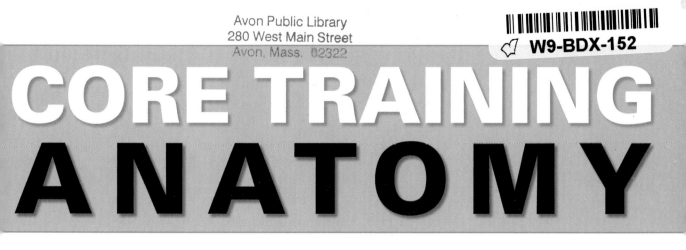

CORE TRAINING
ANATOMY

General Disclaimer

The contents of this book are intended to provide useful information to the general public. All materials, including texts, graphics, and images, are for informational purposes only and are not a substitute for medical diagnosis, advice, or treatment for specific medical conditions. All readers should seek expert medical care and consult their own physicians before commencing any exercise program or for any general or specific health issues. The author and publishers do not recommend or endorse specific treatments, procedures, advice, or other information found in this book and specifically disclaim all responsibility for any and all liability, loss, or risk, personal or otherwise, which is incurred as a consequence, directly or indirectly, of the use or application of any of the material in this publication.

Thunder Bay Press
An imprint of the Baker & Taylor Publishing Group
10350 Barnes Canyon Road, San Diego, CA 92121
www.thunderbaybooks.com

THUNDER BAY
P · R · E · S · S

All notations of errors or omissions should be addressed to Thunder Bay Press, Editorial Department, at the above address. All other correspondence (author inquiries, permissions) concerning the content of this book should be addressed to Moseley Road, Inc., 123 Main Street, Irvington, NY 10533. www.moseleyroad.com.

ISBN-13: 978-1-60710-210-6
ISBN-10: 1-60710-210-2

Printed in Canada

1 2 3 4 5 15 14 13 12 11

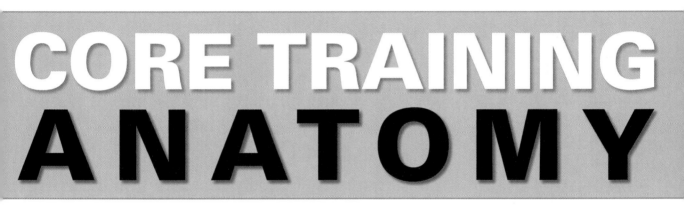

CORE TRAINING ANATOMY

An Insider's Guide to Building a Strong Core

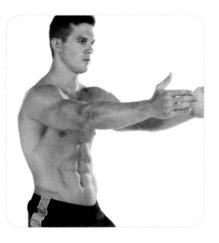

Dr. Abigail Ellsworth

THUNDER BAY
P·R·E·S·S

San Diego, California

CONTENTS

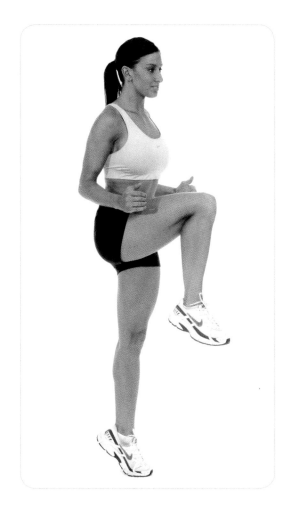

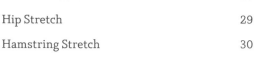

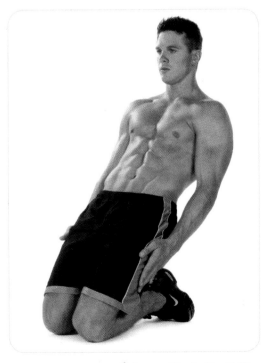

INTRODUCTION: YOUR CORE

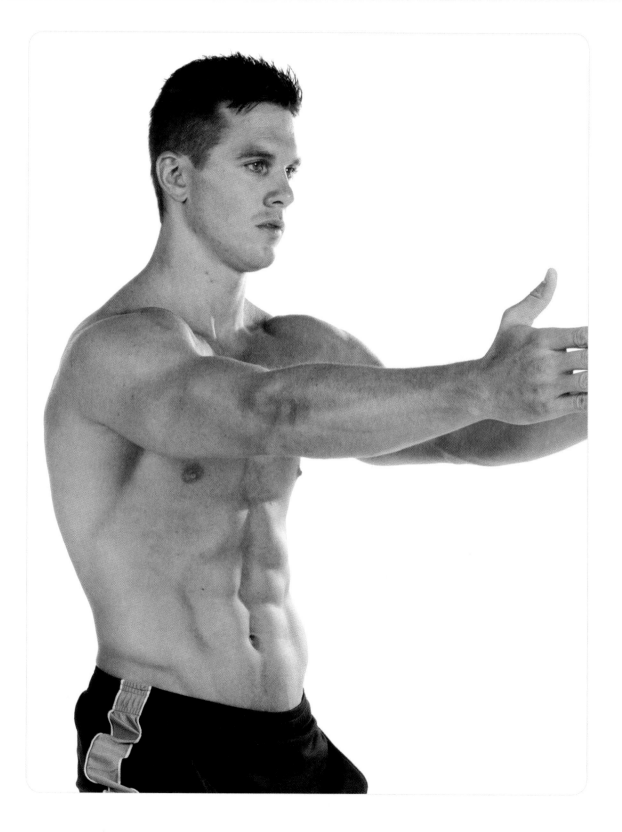

If you've ever taken a fitness class, you've probably heard trainers talking about the "core muscles" of the body. But where are these muscles? What do they do?

The core muscles are the deep muscle layers that lie close to the spine and provide structural support for the entire body. They provide internal pressure to allow intense pushing (such as that during childbirth) or to expel substances (such as vomit, feces, or carbon-laden air). These core muscles are divided into two groups: major core and minor core muscles. The major muscles of the core reside on the trunk and include the belly area and the mid and lower back. This area encompasses the pelvic floor muscles (levator ani, pubococcygeus, iliococcygeus, puborectalis and coccygeus), the abdominals (rectus abdominis, transversus abdominis, obliquus externus, and obliquus internus), the spinal extensors (multifidus spinae, erector spinae, splenius, longissimus thoracis, and semispinalis) and the diaphragm. The minor core muscles include the latissimus dorsi, gluteus maximus, and trapezius (upper, middle, and lower). These minor core muscles assist the major muscles when the body engages in activities or movements that require added stability.

Why is the core so important? Because the functional everyday movements of the body are highly dependent on the core. It stabilizes the trunk and pelvis, allowing the arms and legs to move properly with activity. Lack of core development can result in a predisposition to injury. Here's an analogy: Think about walking on a beach. When you first step on the beach, the sand is loose and deep, and you'll find it really hard to move and walk in. You need to expend a lot of energy and effort. As you progress down toward the water, you'll notice that the sand is now firmer and packed down, making your movement easier and more efficient. Lack of core stability is like trying to walk or run on the top of the beach, where the sand is loose and difficult to move in. While trying to navigate through it, you can easily injure yourself, twisting your ankle, for example. But having a strong core is like walking over firm sand—it's far easier for you to get where you want to go. A strong core makes it easier to move with any activity.

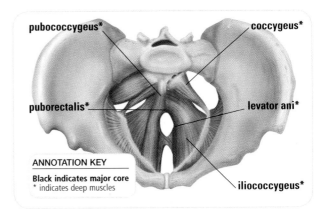

pubococcygeus*

coccygeus*

puborectalis*

levator ani*

ANNOTATION KEY

Black indicates major core
* indicates deep muscles

iliococcygeus*

The way a body moves and the muscles needed to do so is called "biomechanics." The forces applied to the body from the world are what determine how those mechanics are going to be used. The word *force* has many different meanings, but here we are going to generally define "force" as the energy transfer required to travel throughout the body during activity. So if you are running, you exert a

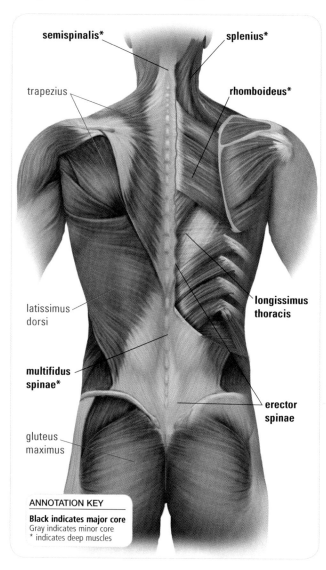

semispinalis*

splenius*

trapezius

rhomboideus*

latissimus
dorsi

longissimus
thoracis

multifidus
spinae*

erector
spinae

gluteus
maximus

ANNOTATION KEY

Black indicates major core
Gray indicates minor core
* indicates deep muscles

strong force on your feet, knees, and hips. The strength of the force decreases the farther away the point of contact is.

In addition to dynamic core function, there is static core functionality. This is the ability of your core to align the bones of your skeleton to resist a force that does not change. What does this mean to you? The static core is what greatly influences your posture. The human body is anatomically designed to take a force (such as that exerted when you sit, walk, run, or jump) and transfer this force through various joints in a desired direction. If your posture and core strength are compromised, then this force cannot be transferred properly, which can lead to injury. Static core strength is one of the hardest forms of core stability to train for and is often overlooked due to the lack of motion. Have you ever noticed how tired you feel after a day of standing at a museum, gazing at art, or standing on the sidelines watching a game? These activities require static core stability, even though you do not feel like you are exerting yourself.

Keeping the core muscles balanced, allowing for equal development and use of the muscles to stabilize, strengthen, and align the body, is crucial to healthy living. It is not just the use of these core muscles, but how they are used that is important. The goal of this book is to teach you how to properly recruit, train, and strengthen these muscles to allow for optimal strength and movement.

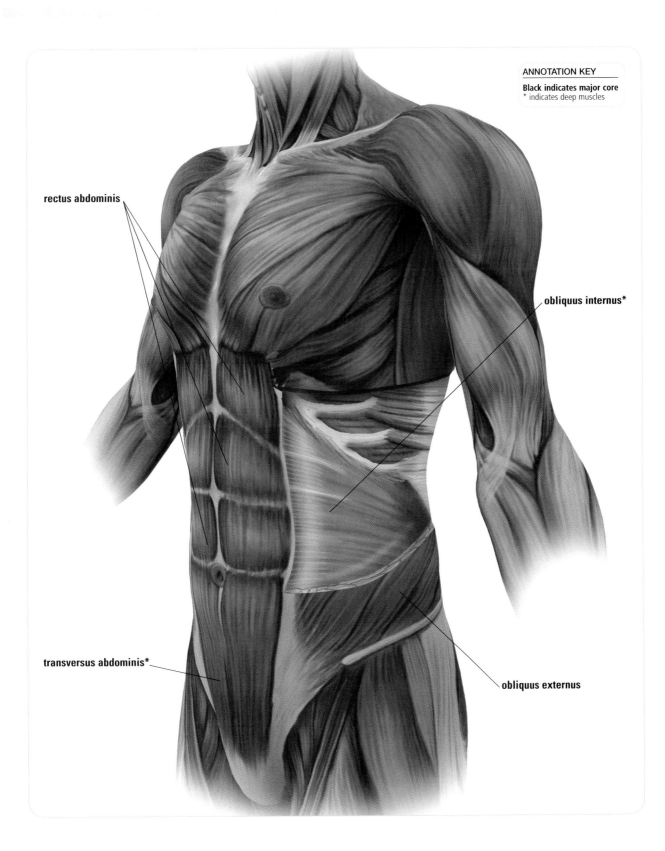

rectus abdominis

obliquus internus*

transversus abdominis*

obliquus externus

NEUTRAL SPINE

What is neutral spine? Why take the time to explain and demonstrate it?

Neutral spine, also known as neutral posture, is one of the most important concepts you need to understand when commencing a core-training regimen. Neutral spine is crucial for ensuring that you properly target and strengthen the muscles of the core, and it also keeps you in a more efficient position for movement. Working in neutral posture is also a component of a holistic approach to movement and exercise in which the body is viewed as an integrated unit, rather than a group of isolated parts. Neutral spine is a key component of both functional exercise and effective core training.

The muscles of the core are closely connected with the postural muscles and the concept of alignment. Neutral posture is the proper alignment of the body between postural extremes. In its natural alignment, the spine is not straight. It has curves in the cervical (neck), thoracic (upper), and lumbar (lower) regions. Neutral alignment helps to cushion the spine from too much stress and strain. Controlling pelvic tilt is one way to begin helping to balance the spine. As certain muscles of the back and abdomen contract, the pelvis rotates. As the pelvis rotates backward, the lumbar curve increases. As the pelvis rotates forward, the curve of the low back straightens.

cervical region

thoracic region

lumbar region

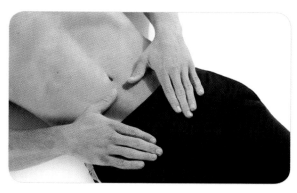

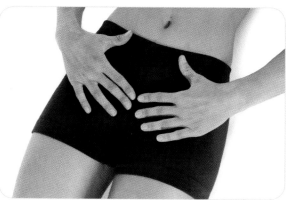

To find your pelvic neutral, place your thumbs on your hip bones and your fingers over your pubic bone, creating a triangle. When you are lying down correctly, with spine neutral, all of the bones will line up on the same plane.

Supine position

Maintaining a neutral spine while you are lying on your back (supine position) is difficult. Pelvic neutral can be found by placing your thumbs on your hip bones and your fingers over the pubic bone (the bone between your legs), creating a triangle. All the bones should line up on the same plane—no tipping back or to one side should be present. The triangle should appear "flat," with all corners on the same plane. This position will prepare you for exercising when you are lying on your back. If you are exercising on your stomach (prone position), however, you can find the neutral spine by pressing your pubic bone into the ground until you feel your back flatten slightly or your stomach lightly lift off the floor. Tuck your chin so that your forehead has contact with the surface, and your neck is now ready for strengthening.

This position not only protects your back and your neck as you exercise, but it also allows you to exercise more productively. Maintaining neutral posture will help decrease the risk of injury and increase the efficiency of movement or exercise.

When people have difficulty achieving or working in neutral posture, it is often an indication of muscular imbalance. Muscular or postural imbalances are a concern because they can lead to injury and chronic anatomical problems or limit performance. Working out of neutral alignment may inhibit the recruitment of certain muscles and make the movements more difficult.

Prone position

FULL-BODY ANATOMY

FRONT

ANNOTATION KEY
* indicates deep muscles

scalenus*

sternocleidomastoideus

pectoralis major

pectoralis minor*

deltoideus anterior

serratus anterior

coracobrachialis*

biceps brachii

rectus abdominis

obliquus internus*

obliquus externus

pronator teres

palmaris longus

flexor digitorum*

flexor carpi ulnaris

extensor carpi radialis

transversus abdominis*

flexor carpi pollicis longus

flexor carpi radialis

tensor fasciae latae

sartorius

iliopsoas*

vastus intermedius*

iliacus*

rectus femoris

pectineus*

vastus lateralis

adductor longus

vastus medialis

gracilis*

tibialis anterior

gastrocnemius

peroneus

soleus

extensor hallucis

extensor digitorum

adductor hallucis

flexor digitorum

BACK

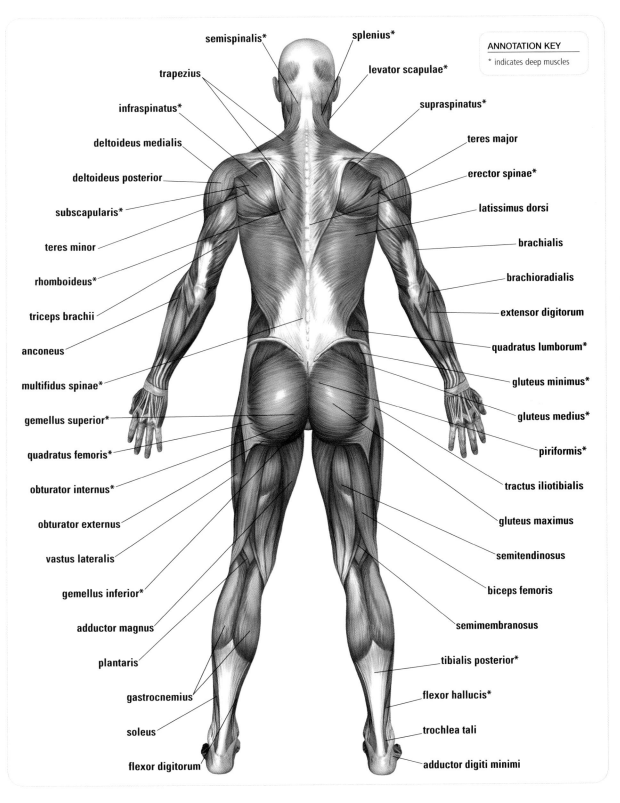

ANNOTATION KEY
* indicates deep muscles

semispinalis*

splenius*

levator scapulae*

trapezius

suprapinatus*

infraspinatus*

teres major

deltoideus medialis

erector spinae*

deltoideus posterior

latissimus dorsi

subscapularis*

brachialis

teres minor

brachioradialis

rhomboideus*

extensor digitorum

triceps brachii

quadratus lumborum*

anconeus

gluteus minimus*

multifidus spinae*

gluteus medius*

gemellus superior*

piriformis*

quadratus femoris*

tractus iliotibialis

obturator internus*

gluteus maximus

obturator externus

semitendinosus

vastus lateralis

biceps femoris

gemellus inferior*

semimembranosus

adductor magnus

tibialis posterior*

plantaris

flexor hallucis*

gastrocnemius

trochlea tali

soleus

adductor digiti minimi

flexor digitorum

STRETCHES

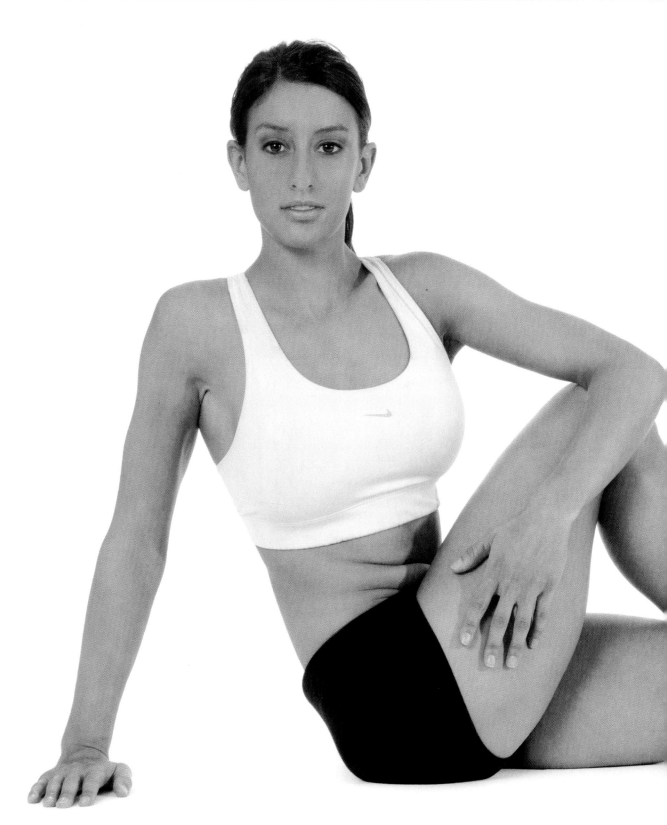

As with any kind of exercise, before beginning a core training regimen, it is important to stretch and warm up your muscles. This preparation will help you avoid injury and optimize your results, guaranteeing an effective and safe workout.

Stretching is most effective after the muscles have heated up a bit, so performing a quick five-minute cardio workout, such as running, jumping rope, bicycling, or rowing, is an ideal way to prepare for these exercises. Then moving on to these warm-up stretches will target the muscles you will be using for your core stability and strengthening workouts.

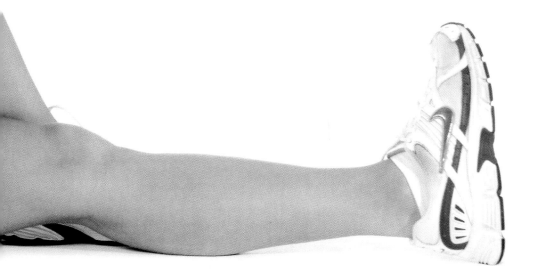

NECK FLEXION

STRETCHES

❶ Placing one hand on your head, slowly pull your chin toward your chest until you feel the stretch in the back of your neck.

❷ Hold for fifteen seconds, and repeat three times.

DO IT RIGHT

LOOK FOR
• Your shoulder muscles to be relaxed.

AVOID
• Pulling too hard with your hand—this is a gentle stretch.

BEST FOR

• splenius
• trapezius

ANNOTATION KEY
Bold text indicates active muscles
Gray text indicates stabilizing muscles
* indicates deep muscles

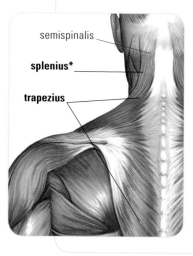

semispinalis

splenius*

trapezius

NECK SIDE BEND

BEST FOR

- scalenus
- sternocleidomastoideus
- trapezius

❶ Gently grasp the side of your head with your hand.

❷ Reach toward the small of your back with your other hand, bending at the elbow.

❸ Tilt your head toward your raised elbow until you feel the stretch in the side of your neck. Hold for fifteen seconds, and repeat three times on each side.

ANNOTATION KEY
Bold text indicates active muscles
* indicates deep muscles

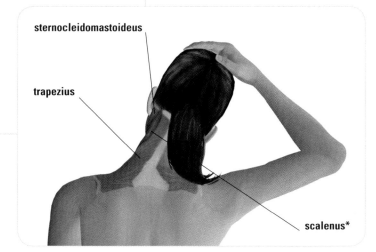

sternocleidomastoideus

trapezius

scalenus*

TRICEPS STRETCH

STRETCHES

❶ While standing, raise your right arm and bend it behind your head.

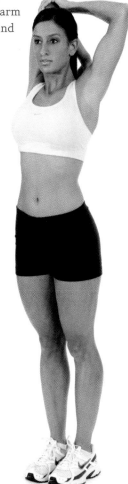

BEST FOR

- triceps brachii
- infraspinatus
- teres major
- teres minor

❷ Keeping your shoulders relaxed, gently pull on the raised elbow with your left hand.

❸ Continue to pull your elbow back until you feel the stretch on the underside of your arm. Hold for fifteen seconds, and repeat three times on each arm.

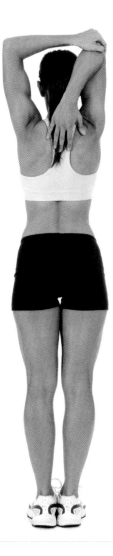

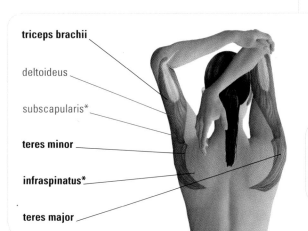

triceps brachii

deltoideus

subscapularis*

teres minor

infraspinatus*

teres major

ANNOTATION KEY

Bold text indicates active muscles

Gray text indicates stabilizing muscles

* indicates deep muscles

LATISSIMUS DORSI STRETCH

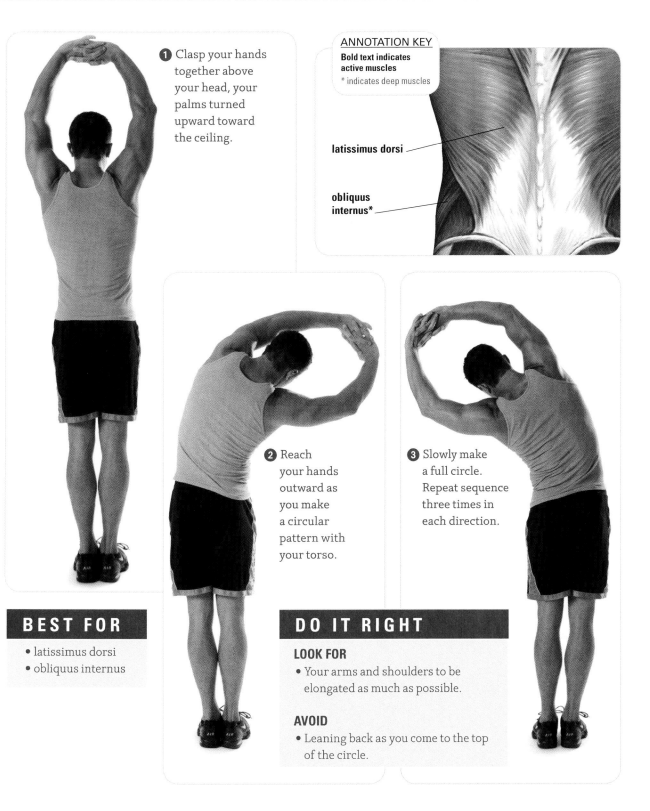

1 Clasp your hands together above your head, your palms turned upward toward the ceiling.

ANNOTATION KEY

Bold text indicates active muscles
* indicates deep muscles

latissimus dorsi

obliquus internus*

2 Reach your hands outward as you make a circular pattern with your torso.

3 Slowly make a full circle. Repeat sequence three times in each direction.

BEST FOR

- latissimus dorsi
- obliquus internus

DO IT RIGHT

LOOK FOR
- Your arms and shoulders to be elongated as much as possible.

AVOID
- Leaning back as you come to the top of the circle.

SHOULDER STRETCH

STRETCHES

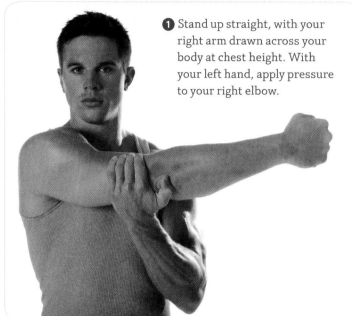

1 Stand up straight, with your right arm drawn across your body at chest height. With your left hand, apply pressure to your right elbow.

BEST FOR

- deltoideus
- triceps brachii
- obliquus externus
- teres minor
- infraspinatus

2 Hold for fifteen seconds, release, and repeat three times. Repeat three times on left arm.

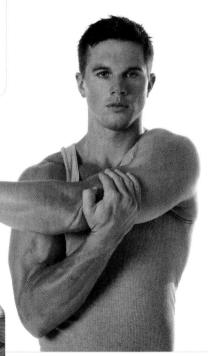

DO IT RIGHT

LOOK FOR
- Your elbow to remain straight while you apply pressure with your hand.

AVOID
- Allowing your shoulders to lift toward your ears.

triceps brachii

deltoideus

infraspinatus*

teres minor

teres major

obliquus externus

ANNOTATION KEY
Bold text indicates active muscles
Gray text indicates stabilizing muscles
* indicates deep muscles

PECTORAL STRETCH

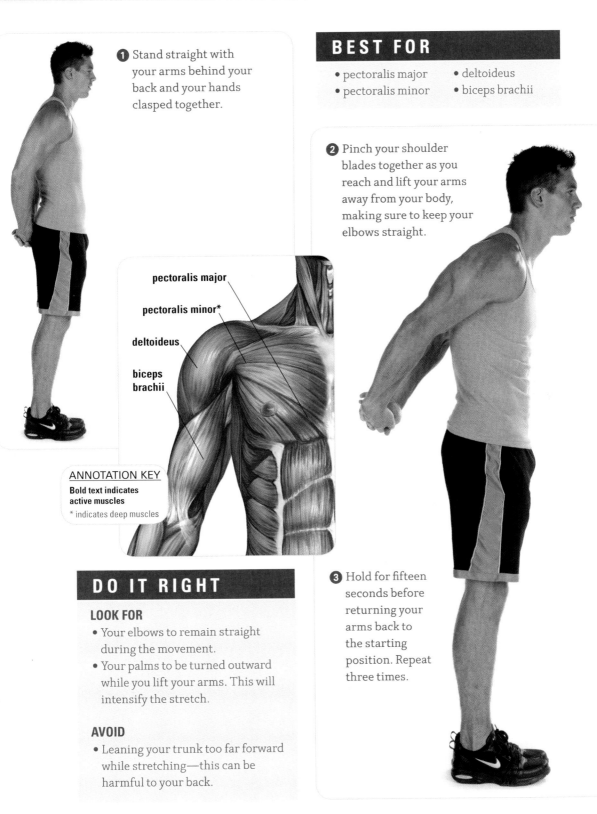

1 Stand straight with your arms behind your back and your hands clasped together.

BEST FOR

- pectoralis major
- pectoralis minor
- deltoideus
- biceps brachii

2 Pinch your shoulder blades together as you reach and lift your arms away from your body, making sure to keep your elbows straight.

pectoralis major

pectoralis minor*

deltoideus

biceps brachii

ANNOTATION KEY
Bold text indicates active muscles
* indicates deep muscles

DO IT RIGHT

LOOK FOR
- Your elbows to remain straight during the movement.
- Your palms to be turned outward while you lift your arms. This will intensify the stretch.

AVOID
- Leaning your trunk too far forward while stretching—this can be harmful to your back.

3 Hold for fifteen seconds before returning your arms back to the starting position. Repeat three times.

QUADRICEPS STRETCH

STRETCHES

DO IT RIGHT

LOOK FOR
• Both knees to remain pressed together.

AVOID
• Leaning forward with your chest.

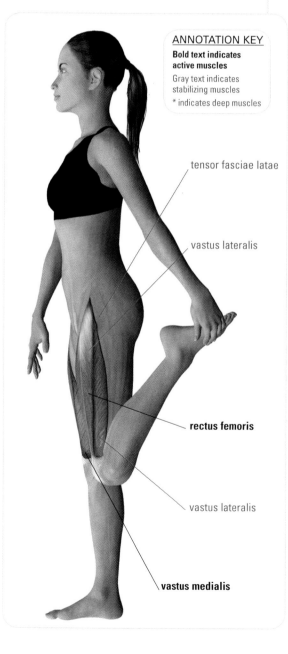

ANNOTATION KEY

**Bold text indicates
active muscles**
Gray text indicates
stabilizing muscles
* indicates deep muscles

tensor fasciae latae

vastus lateralis

rectus femoris

vastus lateralis

vastus medialis

1 Stand with your feet together. Bend your left leg behind you, and grasp your foot with your left hand. Pull your heel toward your buttocks until you feel a stretch in the front of your thigh. Keep both knees together and aligned.

2 Hold for fifteen seconds. Repeat sequence three times on each leg.

BEST FOR

• rectus femoris
• vastus lateralis
• vastus medialis
• vastus intermedius

ILIOTIBIAL BAND STRETCH

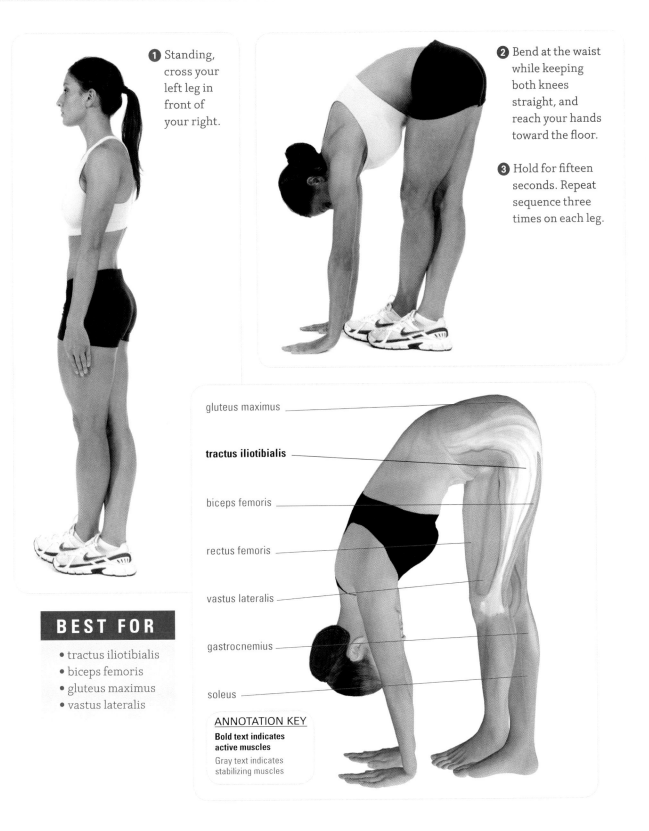

1 Standing, cross your left leg in front of your right.

2 Bend at the waist while keeping both knees straight, and reach your hands toward the floor.

3 Hold for fifteen seconds. Repeat sequence three times on each leg.

gluteus maximus

tractus iliotibialis

biceps femoris

rectus femoris

vastus lateralis

gastrocnemius

soleus

BEST FOR

- tractus iliotibialis
- biceps femoris
- gluteus maximus
- vastus lateralis

ANNOTATION KEY
Bold text indicates active muscles
Gray text indicates stabilizing muscles

ADDUCTOR STRETCH

STRETCHES

1 Standing, separate your feet wider than hip width, so that you are in a straddle position. Bend your knees.

2 Place your hands on your knees and bend at your hips, keeping your spine in neutral and your shoulders slightly forward.

BEST FOR

- adductor longus
- adductor magnus
- peroneus
- biceps femoris
- semitendinosus
- semimembranosus
- piriformis

DO IT RIGHT

LOOK FOR
- Your trunk to remain aligned as you move from side to side.
- Your neck and shoulders to remain relaxed.
- Your hand placement on your thighs to assist your posture.

AVOID
- Rounding your spine.
- Allowing your feet to shift or lift off the floor.
- Allowing your knees to extend over your toes while bending.

3 Keeping your torso in the same position and your hips behind your heels, shift your weight to one side, bending your knee while extending your opposite leg. Hold for ten seconds and repeat on other side.

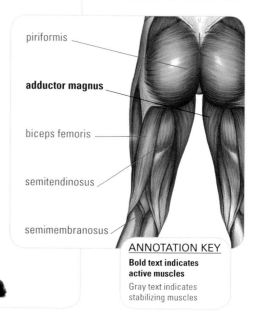

piriformis

adductor magnus

biceps femoris

semitendinosus

semimembranosus

ANNOTATION KEY
Bold text indicates active muscles
Gray text indicates stabilizing muscles

HIP-TO-THIGH STRETCH

1 Kneeling on your left knee, place your right foot on the floor in front of you so that your right knee is bent less than 90 degrees.

2 Bring your torso forward, bending your right knee so that your knee shifts toward your toes. Keeping your torso in neutral position, press your right hip forward and downward to create a stretch over the front of your thigh. Raise your arms up toward the ceiling, keeping your shoulders relaxed.

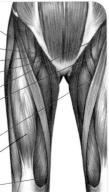

tensor fasciae latae
pectineus*
psoas minor*
iliopsoas*
psoas major*
iliacus*
adductor longus
rectus femoris
gracilis*

ANNOTATION KEY
Bold text indicates active muscles
Gray text indicates stabilizing muscles
* indicates deep muscles

3 Bring your arms down and move your hips backward. Straighten your right leg, and bring your torso forward. Place your hands on either side of your straight leg for support.

4 Hold for ten seconds, and repeat the forward and backward movement five times on each leg.

DO IT RIGHT

LOOK FOR
• Your shoulders and neck to remain relaxed.
• Your entire body to move as one unit as you go into the stretch.

AVOID
• Extending your front knee too far over the planted foot.
• Rotating your hips.
• Shifting the knee of the back leg outward.

MODIFICATION

More difficult: During the backward movement, raise your back knee off the floor and straighten your back leg. Keep your hands on the floor.

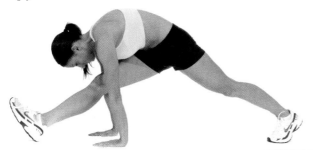

BEST FOR

• iliacus
• iliopsoas
• biceps femoris
• rectus femoris

SPINE STRETCH

STRETCHES

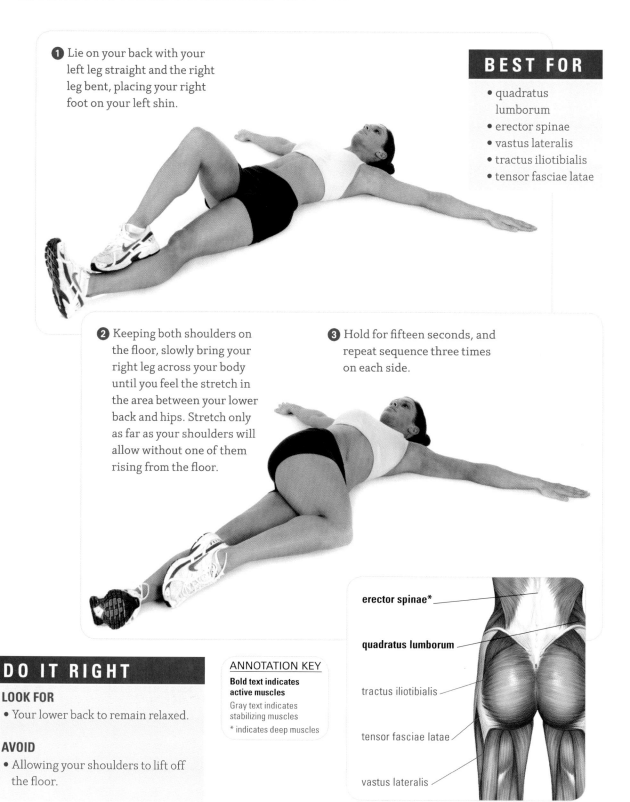

1 Lie on your back with your left leg straight and the right leg bent, placing your right foot on your left shin.

2 Keeping both shoulders on the floor, slowly bring your right leg across your body until you feel the stretch in the area between your lower back and hips. Stretch only as far as your shoulders will allow without one of them rising from the floor.

3 Hold for fifteen seconds, and repeat sequence three times on each side.

DO IT RIGHT

LOOK FOR
- Your lower back to remain relaxed.

AVOID
- Allowing your shoulders to lift off the floor.

ANNOTATION KEY
Bold text indicates active muscles
Gray text indicates stabilizing muscles
* indicates deep muscles

erector spinae*

quadratus lumborum

tractus iliotibialis

tensor fasciae latae

vastus lateralis

LUMBAR STRETCH

1 Lie flat on the floor with both feet and knees together, your knees bent.

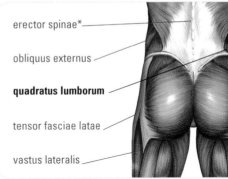

erector spinae*

obliquus externus

quadratus lumborum

tensor fasciae latae

vastus lateralis

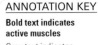

ANNOTATION KEY

Bold text indicates active muscles

Gray text indicates stabilizing muscles

* indicates deep muscles

2 Slowly rock knees from side to side until you feel a stretch along your lower back through the hips or until your knees reach the floor. Repeat ten times.

BEST FOR

- quadratus lumborum
- erector spinae
- obliquus externus

PIRIFORMIS STRETCH

STRETCHES

❶ Lie on your back with your knees bent.

❷ Bring your left ankle over your right knee, resting it on your thigh. Place both hands around your right thigh.

❸ Gently pull your right thigh toward your chest until you feel the stretch in your buttocks. Hold for fifteen seconds and switch sides. Repeat sequence on your left leg.

BEST FOR

• piriformis
• gluteus maximus
• gluteus medius

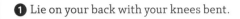

gluteus medius*

piriformis*

gluteus maximus

ANNOTATION KEY

Bold text indicates active muscles

Gray text indicates stabilizing muscles

* indicates deep muscles

HIP STRETCH

1 In a seated position, extend your left leg straight in front of you, and bend your right knee. Cross your bent knee over the straight leg, and keep your foot flat on the ground.

2 Wrap your left arm around the bent knee so that you are able to apply pressure to your leg to rotate your torso. Place your right hand on the floor for stability.

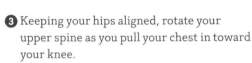

3 Keeping your hips aligned, rotate your upper spine as you pull your chest in toward your knee.

4 Hold for thirty seconds. Slowly release, and repeat five times on each side.

DO IT RIGHT

LOOK FOR
- Your neck and shoulders to remain relaxed.
- Your active hand to apply even pressure to your leg.
- Your torso to remain upright as you pull your knee and torso together.

AVOID
- Rounding your torso.
- Lifting the foot of your bent leg off the floor.
- Straining your neck as you rotate.

ANNOTATION KEY
Bold text indicates active muscles
Gray text indicates stabilizing muscles
* indicates deep muscles

BEST FOR

- obliquus internus
- obliquus externus
- quadratus lumborum
- multifidus spinae
- tractus iliotibialis
- gluteus maximus
- gluteus medius
- piriformis

latissimus dorsi

obliquus internus*

obliquus externus

quadratus lumborum

multifidus spinae*

gluteus medius*

piriformis*

tractus iliotibialis

gluteus maximus

HAMSTRING STRETCH

STRETCHES

1 Lie on your back with both knees bent and your feet flat on the floor.

2 Grasp your left leg behind the knee, and draw your knee in toward your chest.

3 Keeping your knee pulled into your chest, flex your toes and contract your quadriceps, so that you begin to straighten your leg.

4 Release your leg into the stretch, and pull it closer toward your chest. Repeat ten times on each leg.

BEST FOR

- semitendinosus
- semimembranosus
- biceps femoris
- gluteus maximus

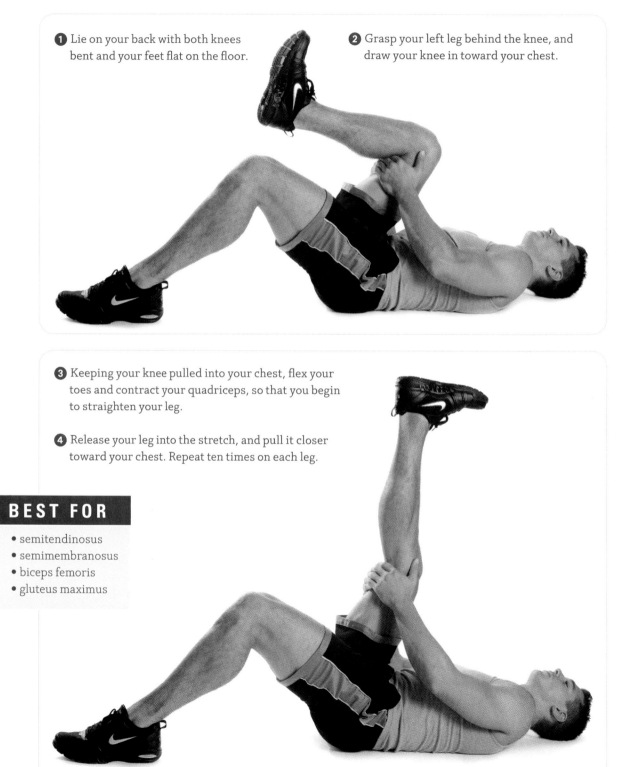

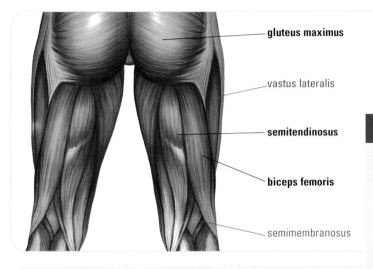

gluteus maximus

vastus lateralis

semitendinosus

biceps femoris

semimembranosus

DO IT RIGHT

LOOK FOR

- Your knee to be pulled in toward the chest throughout the movement.
- Your neck and shoulders to remain relaxed.
- Your toes to be flexed.

AVOID

- Rounding your shoulders and lifting your head.
- Rolling your stabilizing leg out of neutral position.

MODIFICATION

More difficult: Straighten the base leg so that it lies flat on the floor before drawing your other knee to the chest.

CORE STABILITY EXERCISES

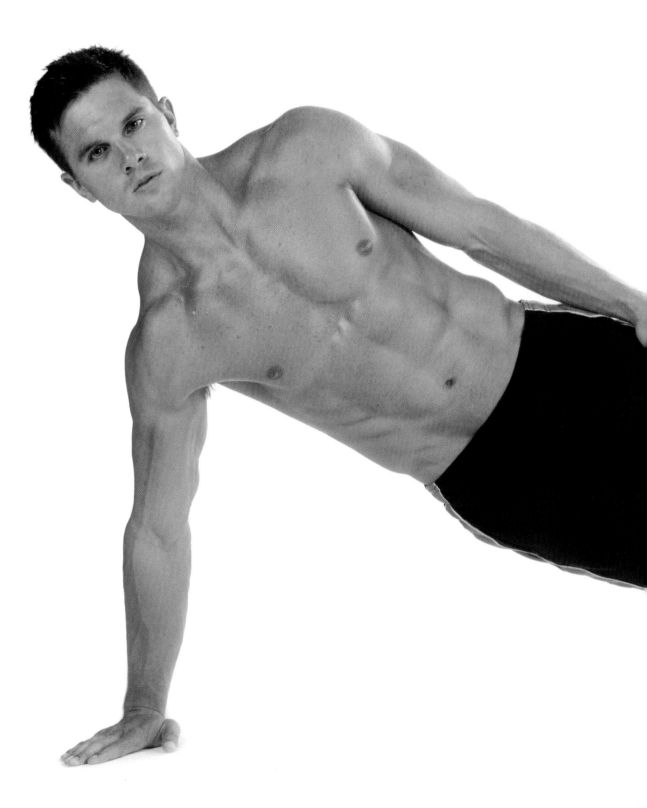

The terms *core stability* and *core strength* are often used interchangeably when discussing the training of core muscles. Yet, core stability and core strength are quite distinct from each other. Training for core stability requires resisting motion at the lumbar spine through the activation of the abdominal musculature and deep stabilizers. This means that the spine does not move with these exercises—the goal is to stay in neutral position. Training for core strength allows for motions to occur through the lumbar spine in an attempt to work the abdominal musculature and deep stabilizers, often in an isolated fashion, as when performing crunches. When strengthening for core stability, you are essentially trying to improve the strength and endurance of the core, as well as gain the muscle control required to perform each exercise correctly.

TINY STEPS

CORE STABILITY

1 Lie in supine position with your knees bent and feet flat on the floor.

2 Place your hands on your hip bones to feel if you are moving your hips from side to side.

3 Raise your right knee to your chest while pulling your navel toward your spine. Hold the position at the top.

BEST FOR

- rectus abdominis
- rectus femoris
- tensor fasciae latae
- gluteus maximus
- transversus abdominis
- obliquus internus

4 As you continue to pull your navel toward your spine, lower your right leg onto the floor while controlling any movement in your hips.

5 Alternate legs to complete the full movement. Repeat six to eight times.

QUICK GUIDE

TARGET
• Lower abdominals

BENEFITS
• Develops lower-abdominal stability, protecting your hips and lower back

NOT ADVISABLE IF YOU HAVE
• Sharp lower-back pain that radiates down the legs

DO IT RIGHT

LOOK FOR
• Your navel to be pulled in toward your spine throughout the exercise.

AVOID
• Allowing your hips to move back and forth while legs are mobilized.

biceps femoris

gluteus maximus

tensor fasciae latae

obliquus internus*

rectus femoris

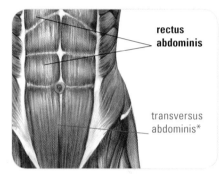

rectus abdominis

transversus abdominis*

ANNOTATION KEY

Bold text indicates active muscles

Gray text indicates stabilizing muscles

* indicates deep muscles

PLANK ROLL-DOWN

CORE STABILITY

DO IT RIGHT

LOOK FOR
- Your spine and legs to remain straight.
- A slow, steady movement.
- Your abdominals to remain up and in.

AVOID
- Bending your knees or spine.
- Allowing your elbows to bend.

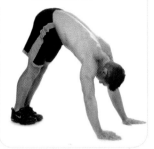

1 Stand tall with your weight equally distributed between your feet.

2 Relaxing your neck, bend from your waist and bring your hands down toward the floor. Place them in front of your feet so that they are flat on the floor.

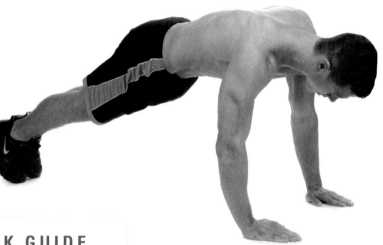

3 Walk your hands away from your feet until your body reaches a plank position, forming a straight line from your shoulders to your heels.

QUICK GUIDE

TARGET
- Pectoral muscles
- Upper-arm muscles

BENEFITS
- Stabilizes core
- Strengthens abdominals

NOT ADVISABLE IF YOU HAVE
- Wrist pain
- Shoulder issues
- Lower-back pain

4 Keeping your arms straight, dip your shoulders three times while maintaining the plank position.

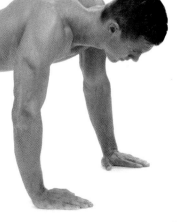

5 Walk your hands back to your feet, and return to an upright position. Repeat ten times at a rapid pace.

MODIFICATION

Easier: Roll down to a plank position on your elbows, rather than on your hands. Supporting your torso with your forearms and maintaining the plank position, dip up and down three times.

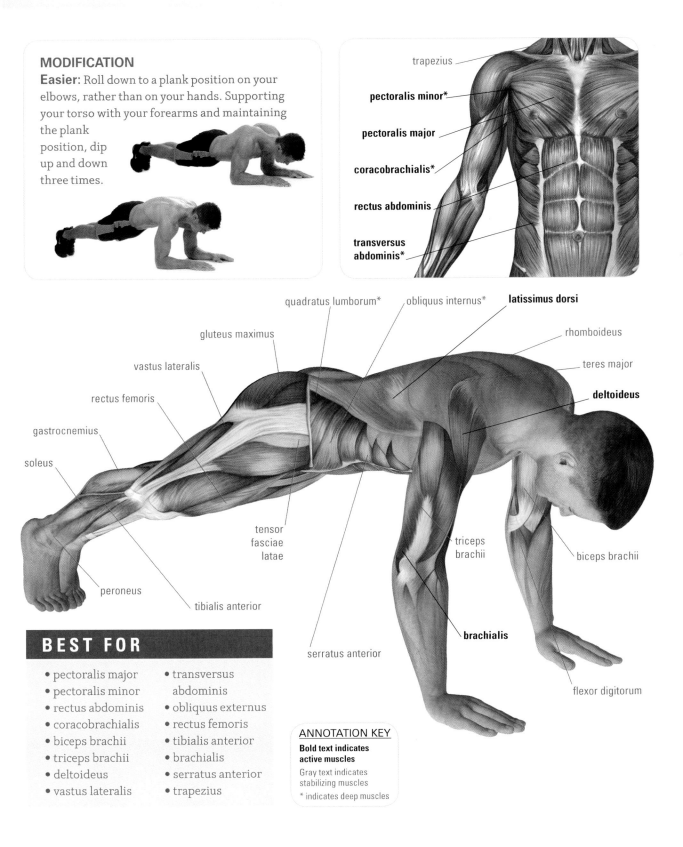

trapezius

pectoralis minor*

pectoralis major

coracobrachialis*

rectus abdominis

transversus abdominis*

quadratus lumborum*

obliquus internus*

latissimus dorsi

rhomboideus

teres major

deltoideus

gluteus maximus

vastus lateralis

rectus femoris

gastrocnemius

soleus

tensor fasciae latae

triceps brachii

biceps brachii

peroneus

tibialis anterior

brachialis

serratus anterior

flexor digitorum

BEST FOR

- pectoralis major
- pectoralis minor
- rectus abdominis
- coracobrachialis
- biceps brachii
- triceps brachii
- deltoideus
- vastus lateralis
- transversus abdominis
- obliquus externus
- rectus femoris
- tibialis anterior
- brachialis
- serratus anterior
- trapezius

ANNOTATION KEY

Bold text indicates active muscles

Gray text indicates stabilizing muscles

* indicates deep muscles

SPINE TWIST

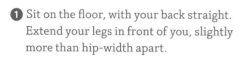

CORE STABILITY

1 Sit on the floor, with your back straight. Extend your legs in front of you, slightly more than hip-width apart.

2 Lift yourself as tall as you can from the base of your spine. Ground your hips into the floor.

QUICK GUIDE

TARGET
• Back flexibility

BENEFITS
• Strengthens and lengthens the torso

NOT ADVISABLE IF YOU HAVE
• Back pain. If your hamstrings are too tight to allow you to sit up straight, place a towel under your buttocks, and bend your knees slightly.

3 Lift up and out of your hips as you pull in your lower abdominals. Twist from your waist to the left, keeping your hips squared and grounded.

4 Slowly return to the center.

DO IT RIGHT

LOOK FOR
• Your torso to rotate along the central axis of your body.
• Your arms to remain parallel to the floor.

AVOID
• Allowing your hips to rise off the floor.

5 Lift up and out of your hips again, twisting in the other direction.

6 Return to the center. Repeat three times in each direction.

BEST FOR

- transversus abdominis
- obliquus externus
- biceps femoris
- gluteus maximus
- tensor fasciae latae
- latissimus dorsi
- teres major
- quadratus lumborum
- deltoideus
- rectus femoris

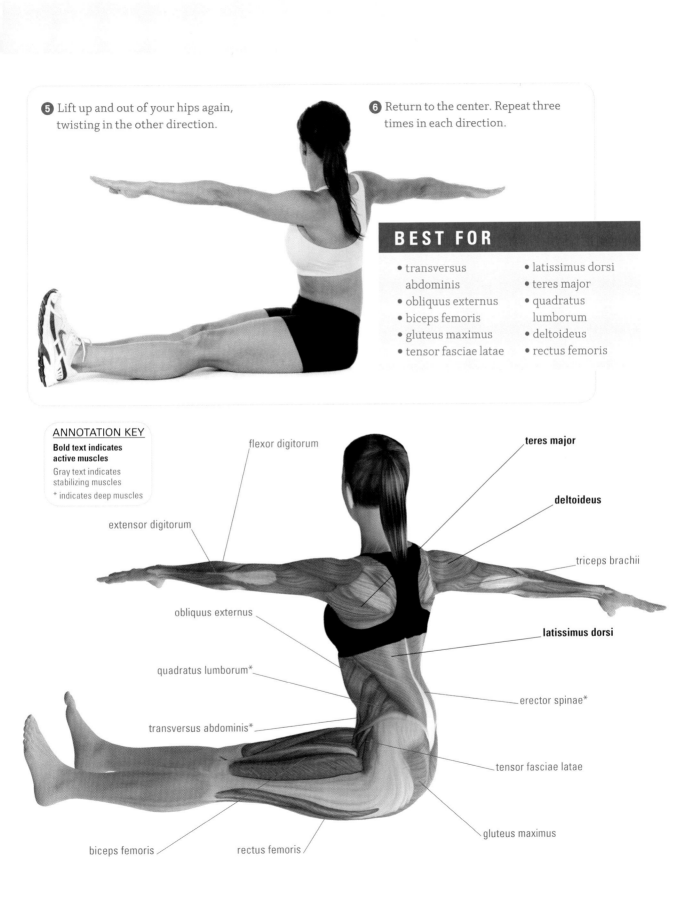

ANNOTATION KEY

Bold text indicates active muscles
Gray text indicates stabilizing muscles
* indicates deep muscles

flexor digitorum

teres major

extensor digitorum

deltoideus

triceps brachii

obliquus externus

latissimus dorsi

quadratus lumborum*

erector spinae*

transversus abdominis*

tensor fasciae latae

biceps femoris

rectus femoris

gluteus maximus

SINGLE-LEG CIRCLES

CORE STABILITY

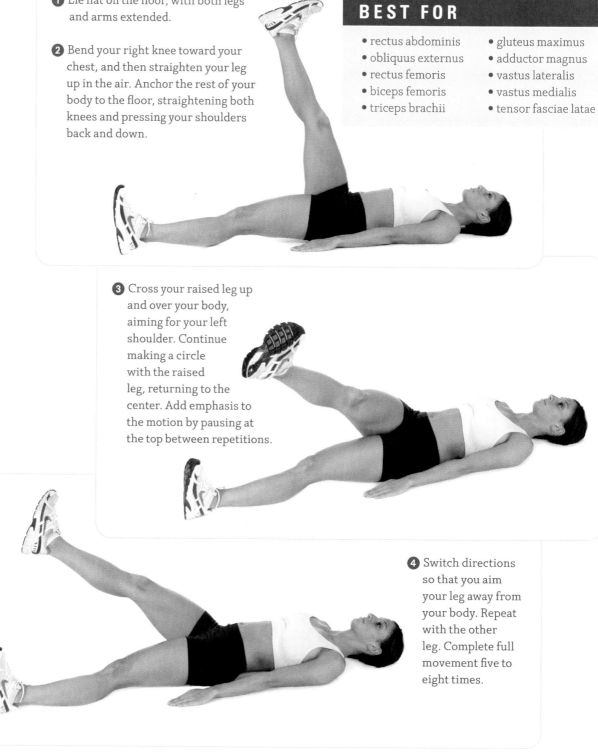

❶ Lie flat on the floor, with both legs and arms extended.

❷ Bend your right knee toward your chest, and then straighten your leg up in the air. Anchor the rest of your body to the floor, straightening both knees and pressing your shoulders back and down.

BEST FOR

- rectus abdominis
- obliquus externus
- rectus femoris
- biceps femoris
- triceps brachii
- gluteus maximus
- adductor magnus
- vastus lateralis
- vastus medialis
- tensor fasciae latae

❸ Cross your raised leg up and over your body, aiming for your left shoulder. Continue making a circle with the raised leg, returning to the center. Add emphasis to the motion by pausing at the top between repetitions.

❹ Switch directions so that you aim your leg away from your body. Repeat with the other leg. Complete full movement five to eight times.

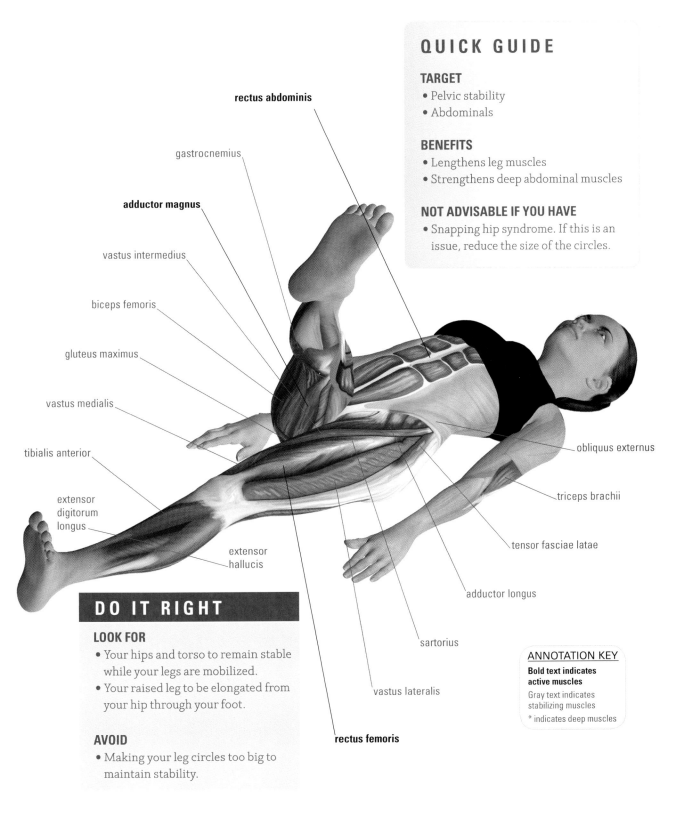

rectus abdominis

gastrocnemius

adductor magnus

vastus intermedius

biceps femoris

gluteus maximus

vastus medialis

tibialis anterior

extensor
digitorum
longus

extensor
hallucis

obliquus externus

triceps brachii

tensor fasciae latae

adductor longus

sartorius

vastus lateralis

rectus femoris

QUICK GUIDE

TARGET
• Pelvic stability
• Abdominals

BENEFITS
• Lengthens leg muscles
• Strengthens deep abdominal muscles

NOT ADVISABLE IF YOU HAVE
• Snapping hip syndrome. If this is an issue, reduce the size of the circles.

DO IT RIGHT

LOOK FOR
• Your hips and torso to remain stable while your legs are mobilized.
• Your raised leg to be elongated from your hip through your foot.

AVOID
• Making your leg circles too big to maintain stability.

ANNOTATION KEY
**Bold text indicates
active muscles**
Gray text indicates
stabilizing muscles
* indicates deep muscles

THIGH ROCK-BACK

CORE STABILITY

1 Kneel with your back straight and your knees hip-width apart on the floor, your arms by your sides. Pull in your abdominals, drawing your navel toward your spine.

2 Lean back, keeping your hips open and aligned with your shoulders, stretching the front of your thighs.

3 Once you have leaned back as far as you can, squeeze your buttocks and slowly bring your body back to the upright position. Repeat four to five times.

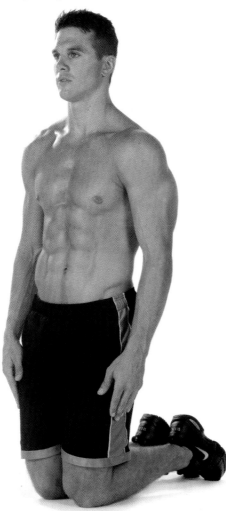

DO IT RIGHT

LOOK FOR
- A straight line to form between your torso and your knees.
- Your abdominals to work to control the movement.
- Your buttocks to be tight.

AVOID
- Rocking so far back that you cannot return to the starting position.
- Bending in your hips.

BEST FOR

- rectus abdominis
- rectus femoris
- vastus intermedius
- vastus medialis
- tensor fasciae latae
- gluteus maximus
- adductor magnus
- sartorius
- biceps femoris
- obliquus internus

QUICK GUIDE

TARGET
- Quadriceps
- Abdominals

BENEFITS
- Stretches thighs
- Strengthens abdominals
- Increases range of motion of anterior ankle

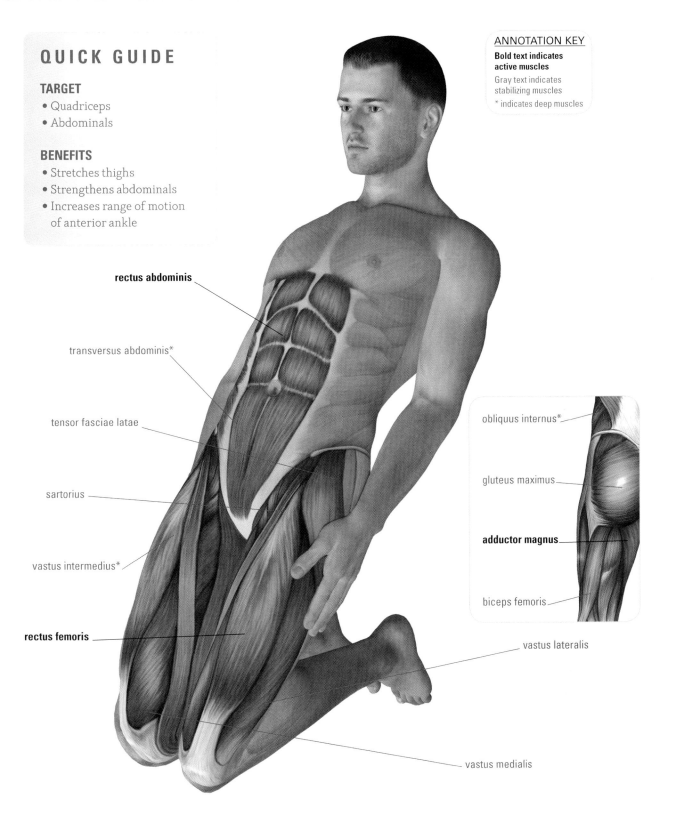

rectus abdominis

transversus abdominis*

tensor fasciae latae

sartorius

vastus intermedius*

rectus femoris

obliquus internus*

gluteus maximus

adductor magnus

biceps femoris

vastus lateralis

vastus medialis

QUADRUPED LEG LIFT

CORE STABILITY

1 Kneeling on all fours, connect with your abdominals by drawing your navel up toward your spine.

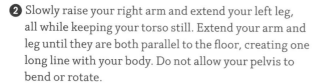

BEST FOR

- gluteus maximus
- biceps femoris
- gluteus medius
- deltoideus
- adductor magnus
- rectus abdominis
- transversus abdominis
- obliquus internus
- tensor fasciae latae
- adductor longus
- rectus femoris

DO IT RIGHT

LOOK FOR
- Your movement to be slow and steady to decrease pelvic rotation.

AVOID
- Tilting your pelvis during the movement—slide your leg along the surface of the floor before lifting.
- Allowing your back to sink into an arched position.

2 Slowly raise your right arm and extend your left leg, all while keeping your torso still. Extend your arm and leg until they are both parallel to the floor, creating one long line with your body. Do not allow your pelvis to bend or rotate.

3 Bring your arm and leg back into the starting position.

4 Repeat sequence on the other side, alternating sides six times.

MODIFICATION

More difficult: Instead of kneeling, press into a plank position to begin, and then raise the opposite arm and leg.

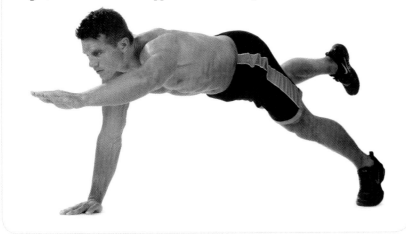

QUICK GUIDE

TARGET
- Core stability
- Pelvic stabilizers
- Hip extensor muscles
- Oblique muscles

BENEFITS
- Tones arms, legs, and abdominals

NOT ADVISABLE IF YOU HAVE
- Wrist pain
- Lower-back pain
- Knee pain while kneeling
- Inability to stabilize the spine while moving limbs

ANNOTATION KEY
Bold text indicates active muscles
Gray text indicates stabilizing muscles
* indicates deep muscles

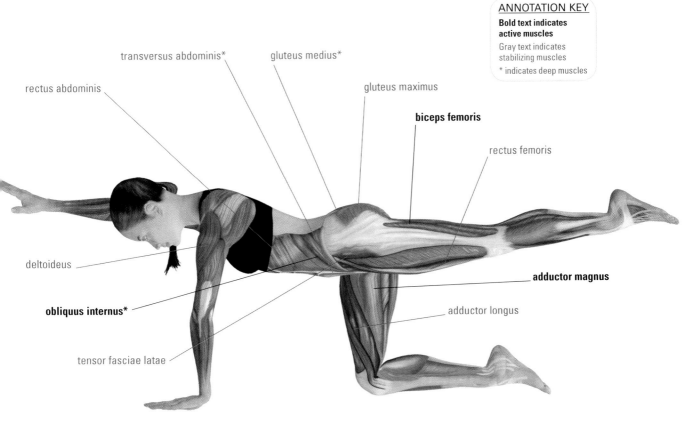

transversus abdominis*

gluteus medius*

gluteus maximus

rectus abdominis

biceps femoris

rectus femoris

deltoideus

adductor magnus

obliquus internus*

adductor longus

tensor fasciae latae

SIDE-BEND PLANK

CORE STABILITY

1 Lie on your right side with one arm supporting your torso, aligning the wrist under your shoulder. Place your left arm on top of your left leg. Your legs should be strongly squeezed together in adduction, with legs parallel and feet flexed. Draw your navel toward your spine.

BEST FOR

- rectus abdominis
- obliquus internus
- obliquus externus
- adductor magnus
- pectoralis major
- pectoralis minor
- triceps brachii
- gluteus medius

QUICK GUIDE

TARGET
- Leg abductors and adductors
- Latissimus dorsi

BENEFITS
- Stabilizes the spine in neutral position with the support of the shoulder girdle

NOT ADVISABLE IF YOU HAVE
- Rotator cuff injury
- Neck issues

2 Press into the palm of your right hand, and lift your hips off the floor, creating a straight line between your heels and head.

3 Slowly lower your hips, returning to the starting position. Repeat sequence five to six times, keeping your legs tight and buttocks squeezed. Repeat on other side.

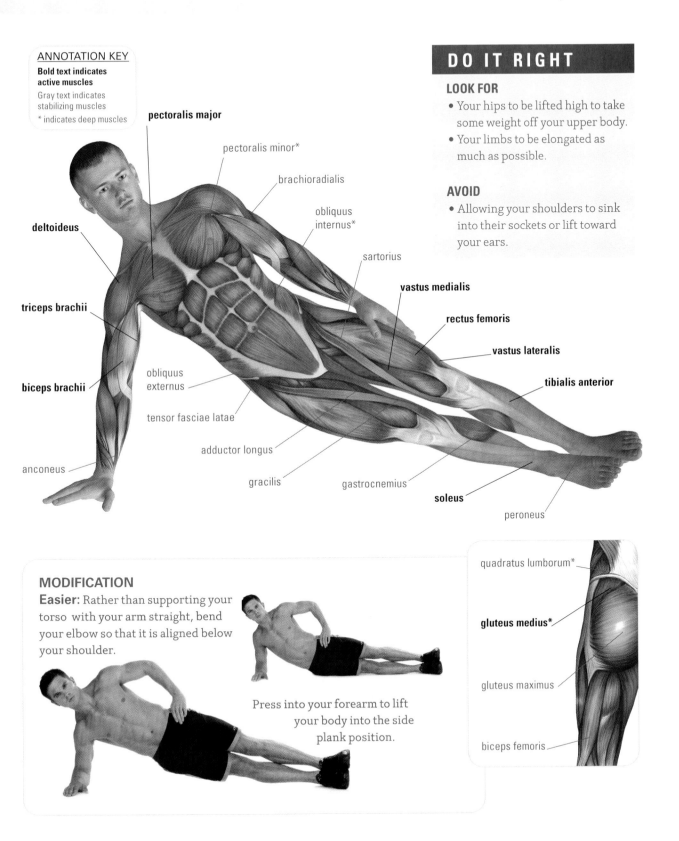

ANNOTATION KEY
Bold text indicates active muscles
Gray text indicates stabilizing muscles
* indicates deep muscles

pectoralis major

pectoralis minor*

brachioradialis

obliquus internus*

sartorius

vastus medialis

rectus femoris

vastus lateralis

tibialis anterior

deltoideus

triceps brachii

biceps brachii

obliquus externus

tensor fasciae latae

adductor longus

gracilis

gastrocnemius

soleus

peroneus

anconeus

DO IT RIGHT

LOOK FOR
• Your hips to be lifted high to take some weight off your upper body.
• Your limbs to be elongated as much as possible.

AVOID
• Allowing your shoulders to sink into their sockets or lift toward your ears.

MODIFICATION
Easier: Rather than supporting your torso with your arm straight, bend your elbow so that it is aligned below your shoulder.

Press into your forearm to lift your body into the side plank position.

quadratus lumborum*

gluteus medius*

gluteus maximus

biceps femoris

HIGH LUNGE

CORE STABILITY

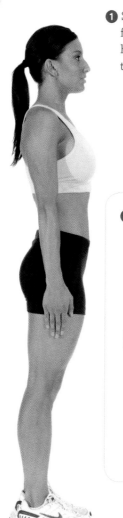

1 Standing tall, move your right foot forward and bend at the hips, bringing your hands down to either side of your foot.

2 Step back with the left foot, keeping your legs in line with your hips. Keep the ball of your right foot in contact with the floor.

3 Press the ball of your right foot on the floor, contract your thigh muscles, and press up to maintain your left leg in a straight position. Hold for five to six seconds.

DO IT RIGHT

LOOK FOR
• Your spine to be lengthened by maintaining the proper position of your shoulders and whole upper body.

AVOID
• Dropping your back-extended knee to the floor.

vastus lateralis

gastrocnemius

plantaris

QUICK GUIDE

TARGET
• Legs
• Abdominals

BENEFITS
• Stretches groins
• Strengthens abdominals, legs, and arms

NOT ADVISABLE IF YOU HAVE
• Hip injury
• High or low blood pressure

BEST FOR

• biceps femoris
• adductor longus
• adductor magnus
• gastrocnemius
• tibialis posterior
• iliopsoas
• biceps femoris
• rectus femoris

4 Slowly return to standing position, and then repeat on the right side. Repeat ten times on each side.

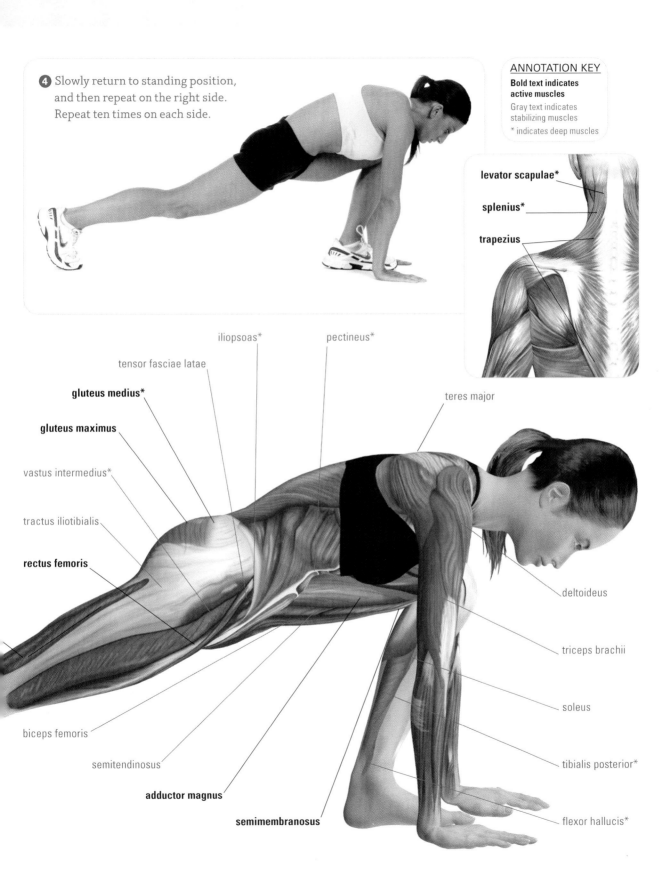

levator scapulae*

splenius*

trapezius

iliopsoas*

pectineus*

tensor fasciae latae

teres major

gluteus medius*

gluteus maximus

vastus intermedius*

tractus iliotibialis

deltoideus

rectus femoris

triceps brachii

soleus

biceps femoris

semitendinosus

tibialis posterior*

adductor magnus

semimembranosus

flexor hallucis*

BRIDGE WITH LEG LIFT

CORE STABILITY

1 Lie in supine position on the floor, your arms by your sides and lengthened toward your feet. Your legs should be bent, with your feet flat on the floor.

2 Lift your hips and spine off the floor, creating one long line from your knees to your shoulders. Keep your weight shifted over your feet.

BEST FOR

- gluteus medius
- gluteus maximus
- rectus abdominis
- transversus abdominis
- quadratus lumborum
- biceps femoris
- iliopsoas
- rectus femoris
- sartorius
- tensor fasciae latae
- pectineus
- adductor longus
- gracilis

3 Keeping your legs bent, bring your left knee toward your chest.

4 Lower your left leg until your toe touches the mat. Be sure to keep your pelvis level.

5 Bring your left knee toward your chest again. Repeat sequence four to five times.

6 Lower your left leg to the floor, switch legs, and repeat the exercise with your right leg. Repeat sequence four to five times.

DO IT RIGHT

LOOK FOR
- Your hips and torso to remain stable throughout the exercise. If necessary, prop yourself up with your hands beneath your hips once you are in the bridge position.
- Your buttocks to remain tightly squeezed as you scoop in your abdominals for stability.

AVOID
- Allowing your back to do the work by extending out of your hips.
- Lifting your hips so high that your weight shifts onto your neck.

QUICK GUIDE

TARGET
- Hip extensor muscles
- Abdominals

BENEFITS
- Improves pelvic and spinal stability
- Increases hip flexor endurance

NOT ADVISABLE IF YOU HAVE
- Neck issues
- Knee injury

ANNOTATION KEY
Bold text indicates active muscles
Gray text indicates stabilizing muscles
* indicates deep muscles

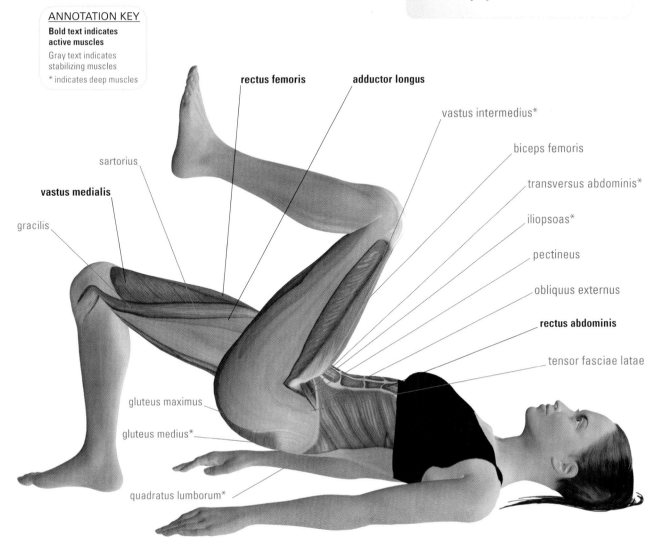

rectus femoris

adductor longus

vastus intermedius*

biceps femoris

transversus abdominis*

iliopsoas*

pectineus

obliquus externus

rectus abdominis

tensor fasciae latae

sartorius

vastus medialis

gracilis

gluteus maximus

gluteus medius*

quadratus lumborum*

PUSH-UP

CORE STABILITY

① Stand straight, inhale, and pull your navel to your spine.

② Exhale as you roll down one vertebra at a time until your hands touch the floor in front of you.

③ Walk your hands out until they are directly beneath your shoulders in the plank position.

④ Inhale, and set your body by drawing your abdominals to your spine. Squeeze your buttocks and legs together and stretch out of your heels, bringing your body into a straight line.

⑤ Exhale and inhale as you bend your elbows and lower your body toward the floor. Then push upward to return to plank position. Keep your elbows close to your body. Repeat eight times.

⑥ Inhale as you lift your hips into the air, and walk your hands back toward your feet. Exhale slowly, rolling up one vertebra at a time into your starting position. Repeat the entire exercise three times.

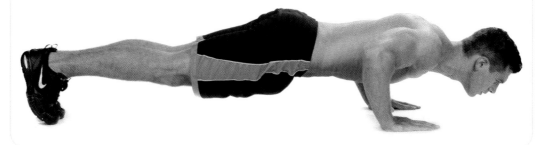

QUICK GUIDE

TARGET
- Pectoral muscles
- Triceps

BENEFITS
- Strengthens the core stabilizers, shoulders, back, buttocks, and pectoral muscles

NOT ADVISABLE IF YOU HAVE
- Shoulder issues
- Wrist pain
- Lower-back pain

DO IT RIGHT

LOOK FOR
- Your neck to remain long and relaxed as you perform the push-up.
- Your buttocks to remain tightly squeezed as you scoop in your abdominals for stability.

AVOID
- Allowing your shoulders to lift toward your ears.

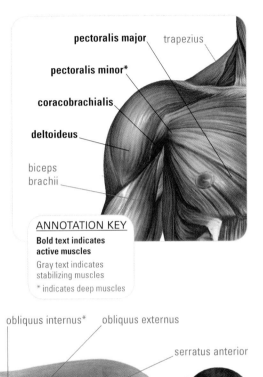

pectoralis major trapezius
pectoralis minor*
coracobrachialis
deltoideus
biceps brachii

ANNOTATION KEY
Bold text indicates active muscles
Gray text indicates stabilizing muscles
* indicates deep muscles

quadratus lumborum*   obliquus internus*   obliquus externus
vastus intermedius*   gluteus maximus   serratus anterior
tibialis anterior
                                                                                rectus abdominis
vastus medialis   extensor digitorum
vastus lateralis   transversus abdominis*
rectus femoris   iliopsoas*

MODIFICATIONS

Easier: Kneel with your hands on the floor in front of you, supporting your torso. Keeping your hips open, bend and straighten your elbows as if you were going to perform a push-up.

More difficult: Place your hands shoulder-width apart on an exercise ball. With the balls of your feet on the floor behind you, complete the push-up movement while maintaining stability on the ball.

More difficult: Place the balls of your feet on top of an exercise ball, while supporting your body with your hands on the floor in front of you. Use your abdominals to keep your body in a straight line and balance as you complete the push-up.

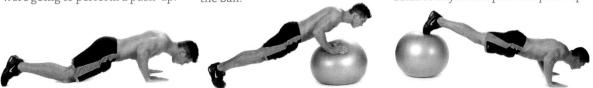

CHAIR DIP

CORE STABILITY

① Sit up tall near the front of a sturdy chair. Place your hands beside your hips, wrapping your fingers over the front edge of the chair.

② Extend your legs in front of you slightly, and place your feet flat on the floor.

DO IT RIGHT

LOOK FOR
- Your body to remain close to the chair.
- Your spine to remain neutral throughout the movement.

AVOID
- Allowing your shoulders to lift toward your ears.
- Moving your feet.
- Rounding your back at your hips.
- Pushing up solely with your feet, rather than using your arm strength.

③ Scoot off the edge of the chair until your knees align directly above your feet and your torso will be able to clear the chair as you dip down.

④ Bending your elbows directly behind you, without splaying them out to the sides, lower your torso until your elbows make a 90-degree angle.

⑤ Press into the chair, raising your body back to the starting position. Repeat fifteen times for two sets.

QUICK GUIDE

TARGET
- Triceps
- Shoulder and core stabilizers

BENEFITS
- Strengthens the shoulder girdle
- Trains the torso to remain stable while the legs and arms are in motion

NOT ADVISABLE IF YOU HAVE
- Shoulder pain
- Wrist pain

BEST FOR

- rectus abdominis
- triceps brachii
- deltoideus
- pectoralis major
- pectoralis minor
- latissimus dorsi

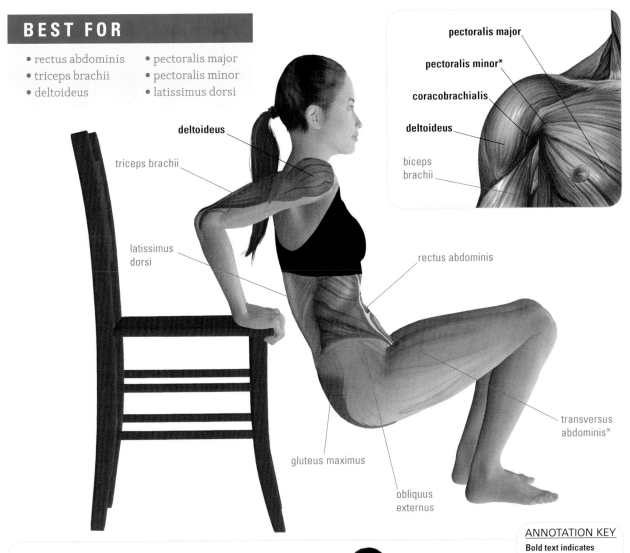

deltoideus

triceps brachii

latissimus dorsi

rectus abdominis

gluteus maximus

obliquus externus

transversus abdominis*

pectoralis major

pectoralis minor*

coracobrachialis

deltoideus

biceps brachii

MODIFICATION
More difficult:

Keeping your knees squeezed together, perform the dips with one leg lifted straight out, parallel to the floor. Repeat fifteen times on each side.

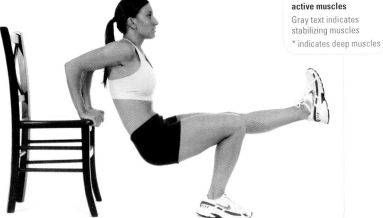

ANNOTATION KEY

Bold text indicates active muscles

Gray text indicates stabilizing muscles

* indicates deep muscles

TOWEL FLY

CORE STABILITY

1 Place a towel on the floor in front of you. Assume the plank position, with your elbows fully extended, and the towel under your hands.

BEST FOR

- deltoideus
- pectoralis major
- pectoralis minor
- coracobrachialis

2 Maintaining a rigid plank position and putting your weight into your heels, move your hands together. The towel should bunch together below your sternum.

3 Straighten out the towel by pressing outward with your arms, returning to the starting position. Repeat ten times.

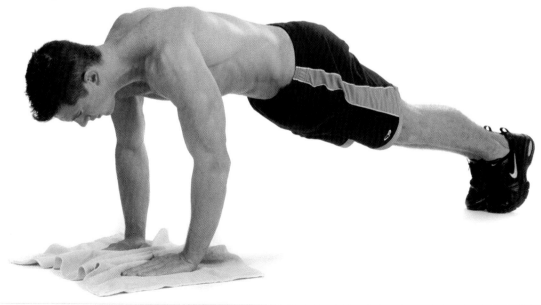

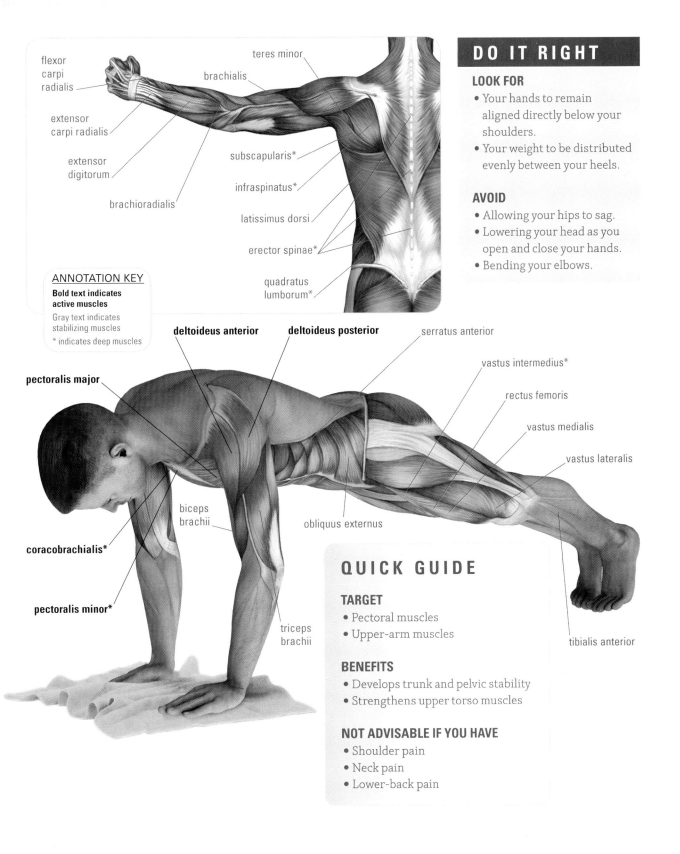

flexor carpi radialis

extensor carpi radialis

extensor digitorum

brachioradialis

teres minor

brachialis

subscapularis*

infraspinatus*

latissimus dorsi

erector spinae*

quadratus lumborum*

ANNOTATION KEY

Bold text indicates active muscles

Gray text indicates stabilizing muscles

* indicates deep muscles

DO IT RIGHT

LOOK FOR
- Your hands to remain aligned directly below your shoulders.
- Your weight to be distributed evenly between your heels.

AVOID
- Allowing your hips to sag.
- Lowering your head as you open and close your hands.
- Bending your elbows.

deltoideus anterior   **deltoideus posterior**   serratus anterior

pectoralis major

vastus intermedius*

rectus femoris

vastus medialis

vastus lateralis

biceps brachii

obliquus externus

coracobrachialis*

pectoralis minor*

triceps brachii

tibialis anterior

QUICK GUIDE

TARGET
- Pectoral muscles
- Upper-arm muscles

BENEFITS
- Develops trunk and pelvic stability
- Strengthens upper torso muscles

NOT ADVISABLE IF YOU HAVE
- Shoulder pain
- Neck pain
- Lower-back pain

HAND-TO-TOE LIFT

CORE STABILITY

1 Stand with both feet equally balanced on the floor, your shoulders relaxed but retracted back. Shift your weight onto your right foot.

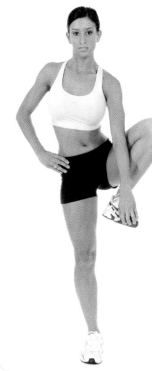

2 Raise your left leg toward your chest by bending your left knee. Grasp your toes with your left hand. Rest your right hand on your right hip.

3 Extend your left leg, straightening it while pulling your foot inward as your extended leg moves to come in line with your torso.

4 Gaze at a single spot on the floor about a body's length in front of you. Flex your foot so that your toes curl back toward you. Hold for five seconds.

5 Lower your foot to the floor, and repeat five times on each side.

BEST FOR

- rectus femoris
- vastus lateralis
- vastus medialis
- pronator teres
- flexor carpi radialis
- palmaris longus
- biceps femoris
- semitendinosus
- semimembranosus
- quadratus lumborum
- piriformis
- gemellus superior
- gemellus inferior
- tibialis anterior
- gracilis
- gluteus maximus

QUICK GUIDE

TARGET
- Leg stability
- Abdominals

BENEFITS
- Strengthens legs and ankles
- Stretches backs of the legs
- Improves sense of balance

NOT ADVISABLE IF YOU HAVE
- Ankle injury
- Lower-back injury

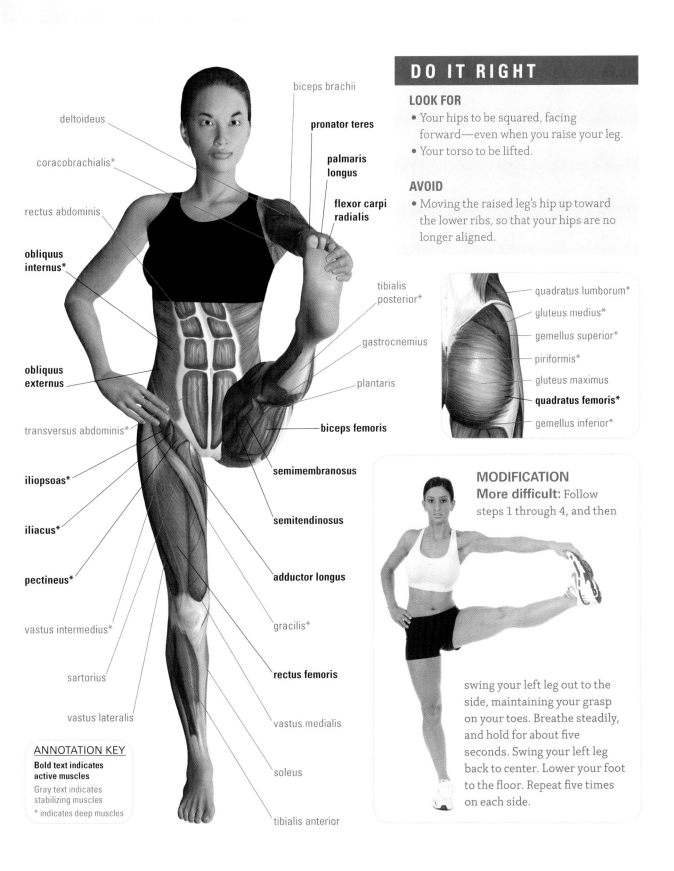

deltoideus

coracobrachialis*

rectus abdominis

**obliquus
internus***

**obliquus
externus**

transversus abdominis*

iliopsoas*

iliacus*

pectineus*

vastus intermedius*

sartorius

vastus lateralis

biceps brachii

pronator teres

**palmaris
longus**

**flexor carpi
radialis**

tibialis
posterior*

gastrocnemius

plantaris

biceps femoris

semimembranosus

semitendinosus

adductor longus

gracilis*

rectus femoris

vastus medialis

soleus

tibialis anterior

DO IT RIGHT

LOOK FOR
- Your hips to be squared, facing forward—even when you raise your leg.
- Your torso to be lifted.

AVOID
- Moving the raised leg's hip up toward the lower ribs, so that your hips are no longer aligned.

quadratus lumborum*

gluteus medius*

gemellus superior*

piriformis*

gluteus maximus

quadratus femoris*

gemellus inferior*

MODIFICATION
More difficult: Follow steps 1 through 4, and then swing your left leg out to the side, maintaining your grasp on your toes. Breathe steadily, and hold for about five seconds. Swing your left leg back to center. Lower your foot to the floor. Repeat five times on each side.

ANNOTATION KEY
Bold text indicates active muscles
Gray text indicates stabilizing muscles
* indicates deep muscles

WALL SITS

CORE STABILITY

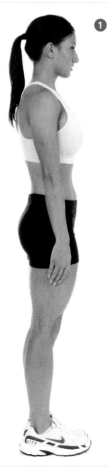

1 Stand with your back facing a wall. Lean against the wall, and walk your feet out from under your body until your lower back rests comfortably against it.

BEST FOR

- vastus medialis
- vastus lateralis
- vastus intermedius
- rectus femoris
- semitendinosus
- semimembranosus
- biceps femoris
- gluteus maximus

2 Slide your torso down the wall, until your hips and knees form 90-degree angles, your thighs parallel to the floor.

3 Raise your arms straight in front of you so that they are parallel to your thighs, and relax the upper torso. Hold for one minute, and repeat five times.

QUICK GUIDE

TARGET
- Quadriceps
- Gluteal muscles

BENEFITS
- Strengthens quadriceps and gluteal muscles
- Trains the body to place weight evenly between the legs

NOT ADVISABLE IF YOU HAVE
- Knee pain

DO IT RIGHT

LOOK FOR
- Your body to remain firm throughout the exercise.
- Your shoulders and neck to remain relaxed.
- Your hips and knees to form 90-degree angles to receive maximum benefit from the exercise.

AVOID
- Sitting below 90 degrees.
- Pushing your back into the wall to hold yourself up.
- Shifting from side to side as you begin to fatigue.

ANNOTATION KEY
Bold text indicates active muscles
Gray text indicates stabilizing muscles
* indicates deep muscles

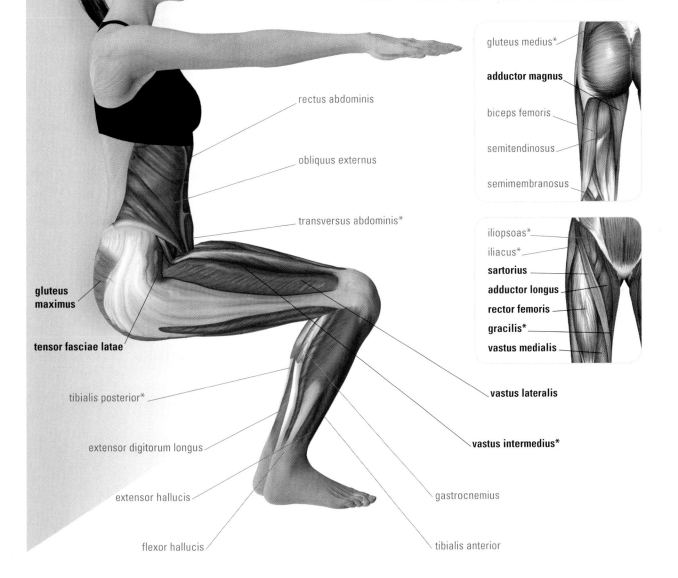

rectus abdominis

obliquus externus

transversus abdominis*

gluteus maximus

tensor fasciae latae

tibialis posterior*

extensor digitorum longus

extensor hallucis

flexor hallucis

gluteus medius*

adductor magnus

biceps femoris

semitendinosus

semimembranosus

iliopsoas*
iliacus*
sartorius
adductor longus
rector femoris
gracilis*
vastus medialis

vastus lateralis

vastus intermedius*

gastrocnemius

tibialis anterior

FRONT PLANK

CORE STABILITY

❶ Sit with your legs parallel and stretched out in front of you. Place your hands behind you with your fingers pointed toward your hips.

QUICK GUIDE

TARGET
• Hip extensor muscles
• Core stabilizers
• Arm muscles
• Leg muscles

NOT ADVISABLE IF YOU HAVE
• Wrist pain
• Knee pain
• Shoulder injury
• Shooting pains down leg

BEST FOR

• gluteus maximus
• biceps femoris
• deltoideus
• rectus femoris
• adductor magnus
• tensor fasciae latae
• rectus abdominis
• transversus abdominis
• adductor longus
• obliquus externus
• latissimus dorsi
• triceps brachii

❷ Press up through your arms and lift your chest up, squeezing your buttocks and lifting your hips while pressing your heels into the floor. Continue lifting your pelvis until your body forms a long line from your shoulders to your feet.

❸ Without allowing your pelvis to drop, raise your right leg, straightened, in the air.

❹ Slowly lower your leg to the floor, and switch to the left leg. Repeat four to six times on each side.

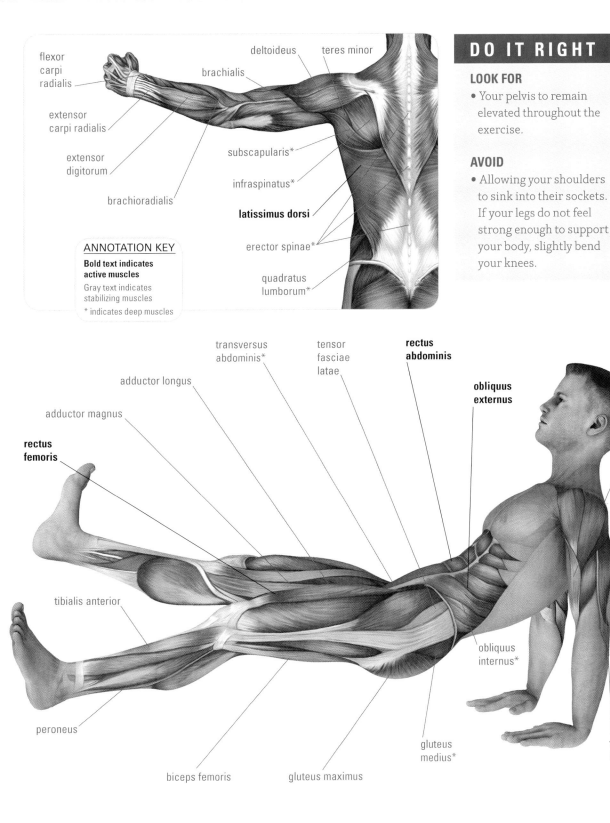

flexor carpi radialis

extensor carpi radialis

extensor digitorum

brachioradialis

deltoideus

brachialis

teres minor

subscapularis*

infraspinatus*

latissimus dorsi

erector spinae*

quadratus lumborum*

ANNOTATION KEY

Bold text indicates active muscles

Gray text indicates stabilizing muscles

* indicates deep muscles

DO IT RIGHT

LOOK FOR
• Your pelvis to remain elevated throughout the exercise.

AVOID
• Allowing your shoulders to sink into their sockets. If your legs do not feel strong enough to support your body, slightly bend your knees.

transversus abdominis*

adductor longus

adductor magnus

rectus femoris

tibialis anterior

peroneus

biceps femoris

gluteus maximus

gluteus medius*

tensor fasciae latae

rectus abdominis

obliquus externus

biceps brachii

obliquus internus*

triceps brachii

SCISSORS

CORE STABILITY

1. Lie with your back on the floor, your arms by your sides and your legs raised in a tabletop position. Inhale, drawing in your abdominals.

2. Reach your legs straight up, and lift your head and shoulders off the floor. Hold the position while lengthening your legs.

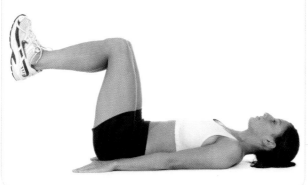

BEST FOR

- biceps femoris
- rectus femoris
- tensor fasciae latae
- rectus abdominis
- obliquus externus
- deltoideus

DO IT RIGHT

LOOK FOR
- Your legs to be as straight as possible.
- Your navel to be drawn into your spine.

AVOID
- Bending your leg.

3. Stretching your right leg away from your body, raise your left leg toward your trunk. Hold your left calf with your hands, pulsing twice while keeping your shoulders down.

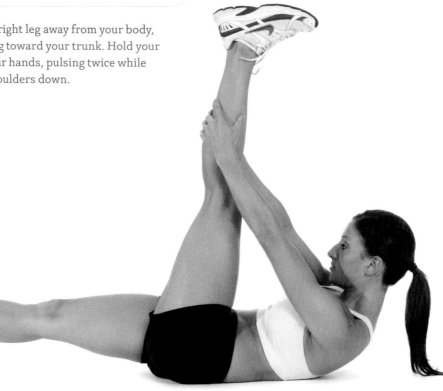

QUICK GUIDE

TARGET
• Abdominals

BENEFITS
• Increases stability with unilateral movement
• Increases abdominal strength and endurance

NOT ADVISABLE IF YOU HAVE
• Tight hamstrings. If this is an issue, you may bend the knee that is moving toward your chest.

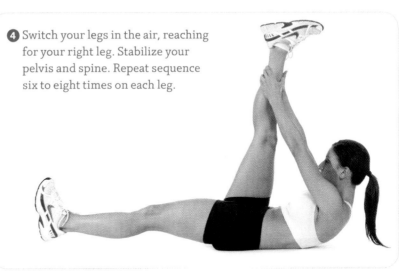

❹ Switch your legs in the air, reaching for your right leg. Stabilize your pelvis and spine. Repeat sequence six to eight times on each leg.

ANNOTATION KEY
Bold text indicates active muscles
Gray text indicates stabilizing muscles
* indicates deep muscles

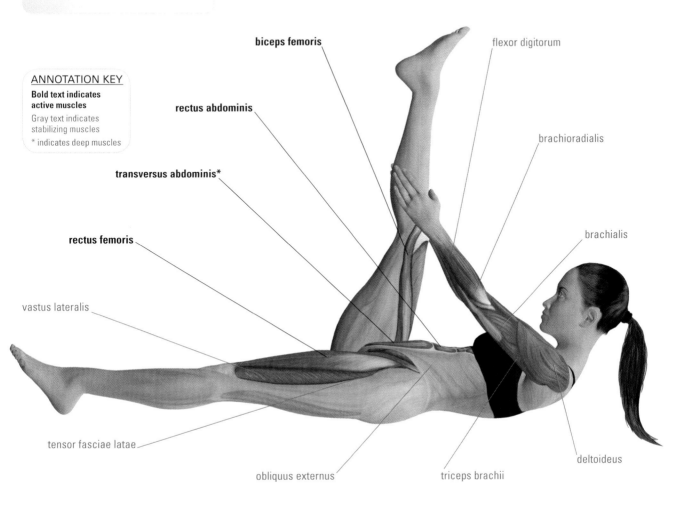

biceps femoris

flexor digitorum

rectus abdominis

brachioradialis

transversus abdominis*

brachialis

rectus femoris

vastus lateralis

tensor fasciae latae

obliquus externus

triceps brachii

deltoideus

SWIMMING

CORE STABILITY

1 Lie prone on the floor with your legs hip-width apart. Stretch your arms beside your ears on the floor. Engage your pelvic floor, and draw your navel into your spine.

2 Extend through your upper back as you lift your left arm and right leg simultaneously. Lift your head and shoulders off the floor.

3 Lower your arm and leg to the starting position, maintaining a stretch in your limbs throughout.

4 Extend your right arm and left leg off the floor, lengthening and lifting your head and shoulders.

5 Elongate your limbs as you return to the starting position. Repeat six to eight times.

QUICK GUIDE

TARGET
• Spinal extensors
• Hip extensors

BENEFITS
• Strengthens hip and spine extensors
• Challenges stabilization of the spine against rotation

NOT ADVISABLE IF YOU HAVE
• Lower-back pain
• Extreme curvature of the upper spine
• Curvature of the lower spine

BEST FOR
• gluteus maximus
• biceps femoris
• erector spinae
• quadratus lumborum
• rhomboideus
• latissimus dorsi

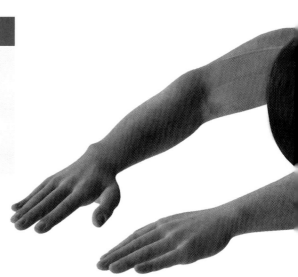

MODIFICATION
More difficult: Instead of lifting the opposite leg and arm, lift both arms and legs simultaneously, continuing to draw your navel into your spine. This version of the exercise is commonly known as the Superman.

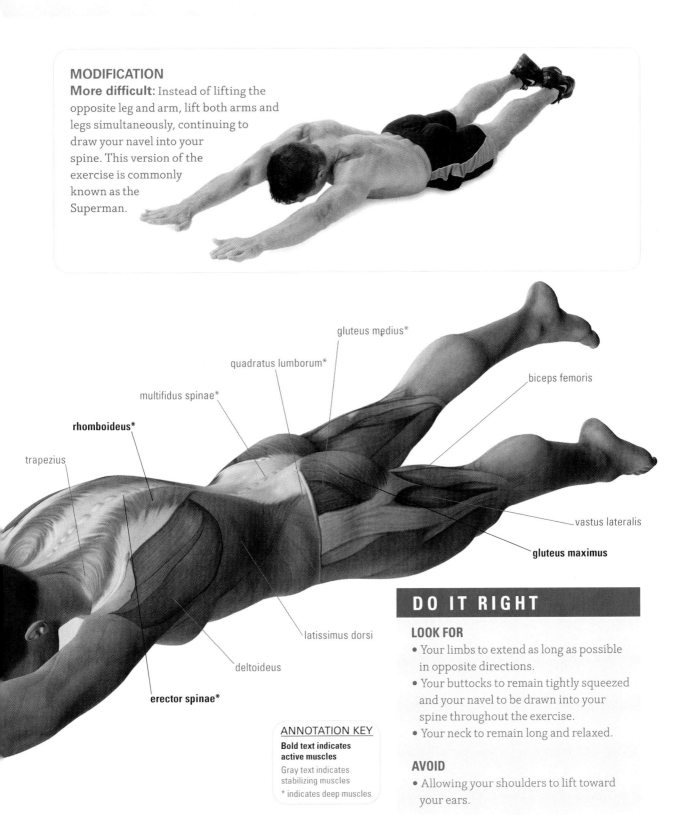

gluteus medius*

quadratus lumborum*

multifidus spinae*

rhomboideus*

trapezius

biceps femoris

vastus lateralis

gluteus maximus

latissimus dorsi

deltoideus

erector spinae*

ANNOTATION KEY
**Bold text indicates
active muscles**
Gray text indicates
stabilizing muscles
* indicates deep muscles

DO IT RIGHT

LOOK FOR
- Your limbs to extend as long as possible in opposite directions.
- Your buttocks to remain tightly squeezed and your navel to be drawn into your spine throughout the exercise.
- Your neck to remain long and relaxed.

AVOID
- Allowing your shoulders to lift toward your ears.

DOUBLE-LEG AB PRESS

CORE STABILITY

❶ Lie on your back with your knees and feet lifted in tabletop position, your thighs making a 90-degree angle with your upper body. Place your hands on the front of your knees, your fingers facing upward, one palm on each leg.

DO IT RIGHT

LOOK FOR
- Your elbows to be pulled in toward your sides.
- Your shoulders and neck to remain relaxed.
- Your feet to be flexed and your knees pressed together.
- Your tailbone to be tucked up toward the ceiling.

AVOID
- Holding your breath while performing the exercise.

❷ Flex your feet and, keeping your elbows bent and pulled into your sides, press your hands into your knees. Create resistance by pushing back against your hands with your knees. Hold for one minute, and repeat five times.

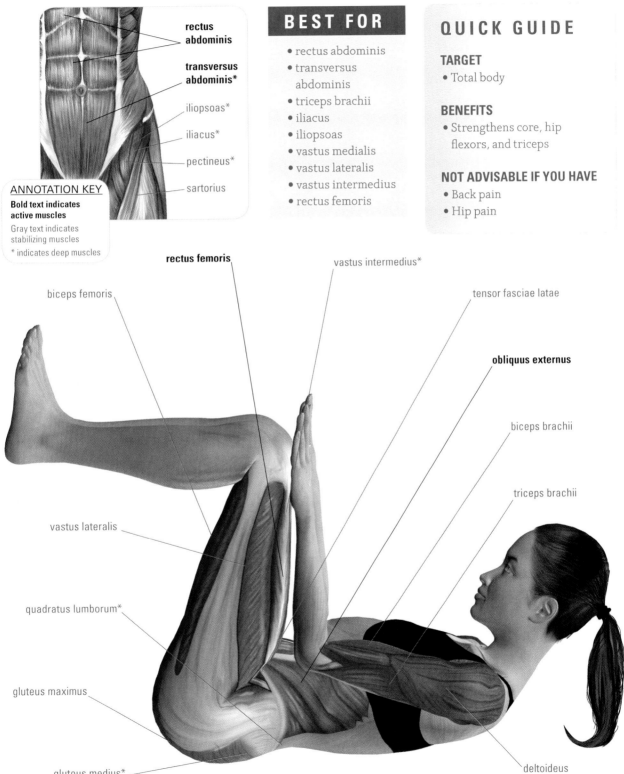

rectus
abdominis

transversus
abdominis*

iliopsoas*

iliacus*

pectineus*

sartorius

ANNOTATION KEY
**Bold text indicates
active muscles**
Gray text indicates
stabilizing muscles
* indicates deep muscles

BEST FOR
- rectus abdominis
- transversus
  abdominis
- triceps brachii
- iliacus
- iliopsoas
- vastus medialis
- vastus lateralis
- vastus intermedius
- rectus femoris

QUICK GUIDE

TARGET
- Total body

BENEFITS
- Strengthens core, hip
  flexors, and triceps

NOT ADVISABLE IF YOU HAVE
- Back pain
- Hip pain

rectus femoris

vastus intermedius*

tensor fasciae latae

biceps femoris

obliquus externus

biceps brachii

triceps brachii

vastus lateralis

quadratus lumborum*

gluteus maximus

gluteus medius*

deltoideus

CLAMSHELL SERIES

CORE STABILITY

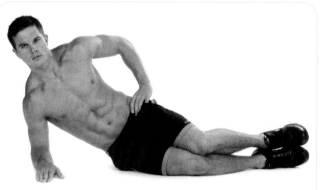

1 Lie on your right side with knees bent and stacked on top of each other. Bend your left elbow, placing it directly underneath your shoulder so that your forearm is supporting your upper body. Place your left hand on your hip.

DO IT RIGHT

LOOK FOR
- Your hips to be stacked and pulled forward slightly.
- Your shoulder and forearm to press into the floor throughout the exercise.
- Your neck and shoulders to be relaxed.

AVOID
- Allowing your hips to move while lifting your knee.

2 Without moving your hips, open your left knee upward, and then return to the starting position. Repeat ten times.

3 Lift both ankles off the floor, making sure to maintain a straight line with the torso.

4 While your ankles are still lifted, lift and lower your left knee to open and close your legs. Repeat ten times.

BEST FOR

- rectus abdominis
- obliquus internus
- obliquus externus
- tensor fasciae latae
- adductor magnus
- adductor longus
- iliopsoas
- iliacus
- gluteus medius
- quadratus lumborum

QUICK GUIDE

TARGET
- Abdominals
- Abductor and adductor muscles
- Rotator cuff

BENEFITS
- Improves pelvic stability
- Strengthens abductor muscles
- Targets the shoulder stabilizers for strengthening and endurance

NOT ADVISABLE IF YOU HAVE
- Shoulder injury
- Lower-back pain

5 The final part of this series begins with both ankles elevated. Lift your left knee to separate your legs, and then straighten your left leg, being careful not to move the position of your thigh. Bend your knee and return to the starting position. Repeat ten times, switch sides, and start from the beginning.

ANNOTATION KEY
Bold text indicates active muscles
Gray text indicates stabilizing muscles
* indicates deep muscles

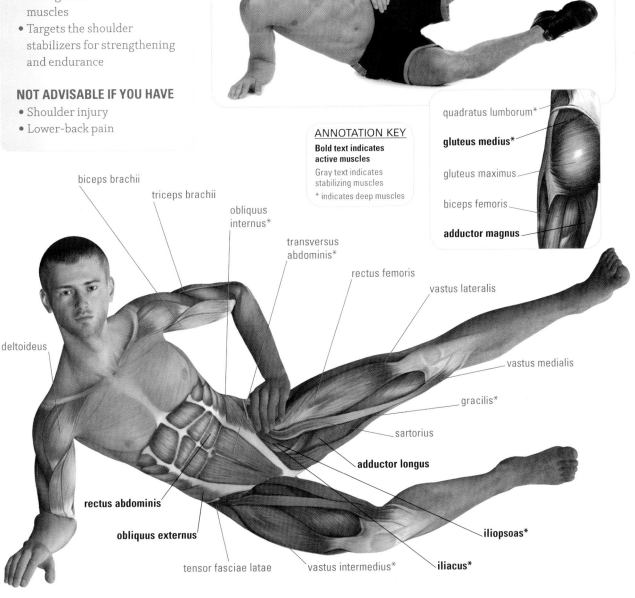

quadratus lumborum*
gluteus medius*
gluteus maximus
biceps femoris
adductor magnus

biceps brachii
triceps brachii
obliquus internus*
transversus abdominis*
rectus femoris
vastus lateralis
deltoideus
vastus medialis
gracilis*
sartorius
adductor longus
rectus abdominis
obliquus externus
iliopsoas*
tensor fasciae latae
vastus intermedius*
iliacus*

PRONE HEEL BEATS

CORE STABILITY

1 Lie facedown with your arms lifted off the floor by your hips, palms up. Draw your shoulders down away from your ears. Turn your legs out from the top of your hips and pull your inner thighs together.

2 Pull your navel off the mat and toward your spine, pressing your pubic bone into the mat. Lengthen your legs and lift them off the mat, tightening your thigh muscles.

DO IT RIGHT

LOOK FOR
- Your buttocks and your abdominals to be squeezed while beating your heels.
- Your breathing to remain steady.

AVOID
- Tensing your shoulders.

ANNOTATION KEY
Bold text indicates active muscles
Gray text indicates stabilizing muscles
* indicates deep muscles

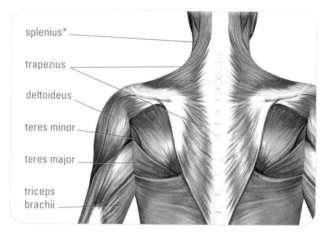

splenius*
trapezius
deltoideus
teres minor
teres major
triceps brachii

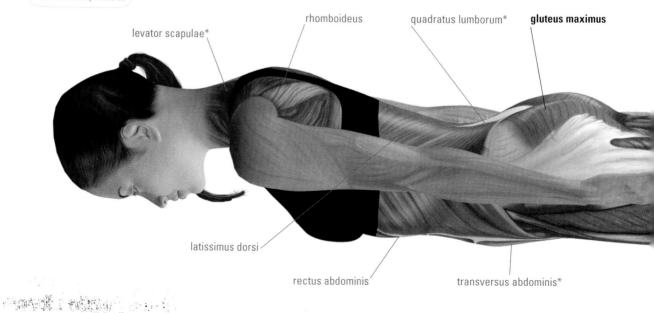

levator scapulae*
rhomboideus
quadratus lumborum*
gluteus maximus
latissimus dorsi
rectus abdominis
transversus abdominis*

3 Press your heels together and then separate them in a rapid but controlled motion.

BEST FOR

- trapezius
- latissimus dorsi
- teres major
- teres minor
- deltoideus
- gluteus maximus
- biceps femoris
- adductor magnus
- soleus
- vastus lateralis

4 Beat heels together for eight counts, then return to the starting position. Repeat sequence six to eight times.

QUICK GUIDE

TARGET
- Core stabilizers

BENEFITS
- Encourages muscles from the entire body to work together
- Lengthens extension muscles

NOT ADVISABLE IF YOU HAVE
- Back pain

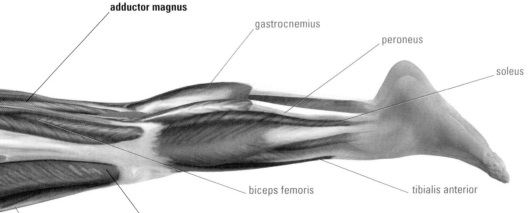

adductor magnus

gastrocnemius

peroneus

soleus

biceps femoris

tibialis anterior

vastus lateralis

rectus femoris

CORE STRENGTH EXERCISES

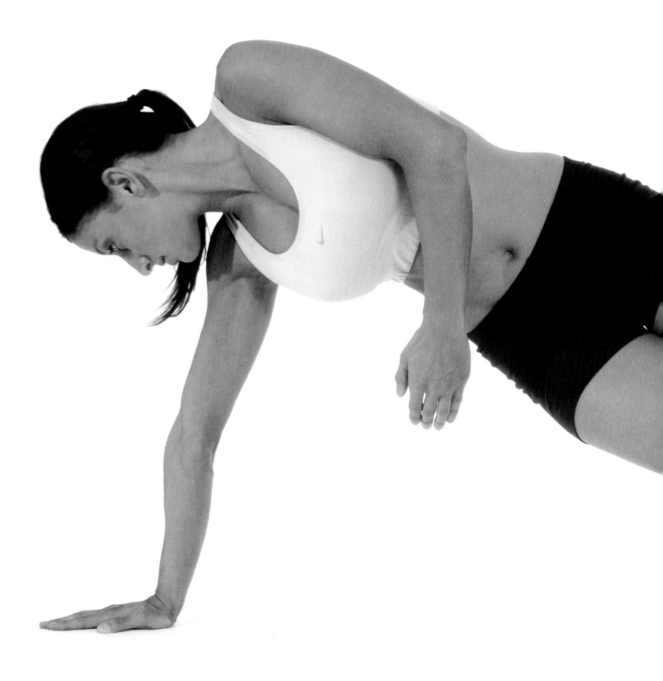

Now that you have mastered core stability, it is time to put the body to work and strengthen it.

Core strength is the balanced development of both the deep and superficial muscles that stabilize, align, and move the trunk of the body. Although these muscles play various roles in the body, their major function is to provide support for your spine. If your core is weak, you are more susceptible to injury—a weak core places strain on your spine and your entire body. Core strengthening stabilizes the muscles of your midsection, including the hips and pelvis, so movements such as running or walking are improved, making it easier to perform activities.

BASIC CRUNCH

CORE STRENGTH

1 Lie supine on the floor with your knees bent, and clasp your hands behind your head.

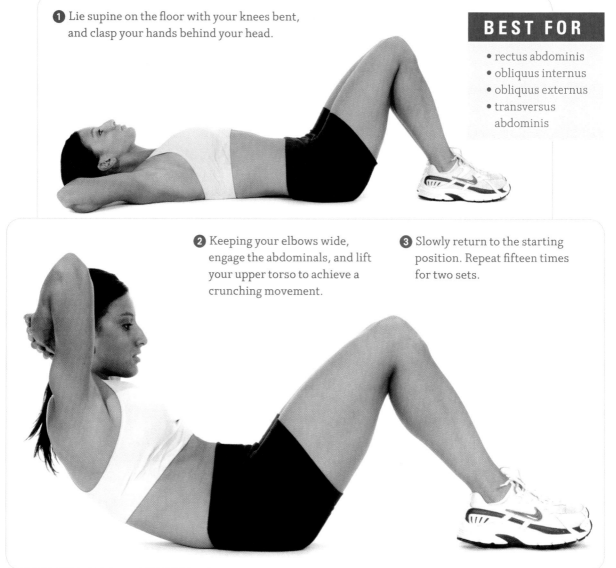

2 Keeping your elbows wide, engage the abdominals, and lift your upper torso to achieve a crunching movement.

3 Slowly return to the starting position. Repeat fifteen times for two sets.

MODIFICATION

More difficult: Begin by lying supine on the floor with your legs outstretched, and your arms over your head. Without lifting your legs, lift your arms and torso in a controlled movement. Continue to curl forward and grasp your feet.

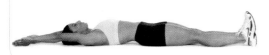
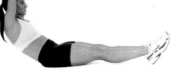
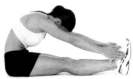

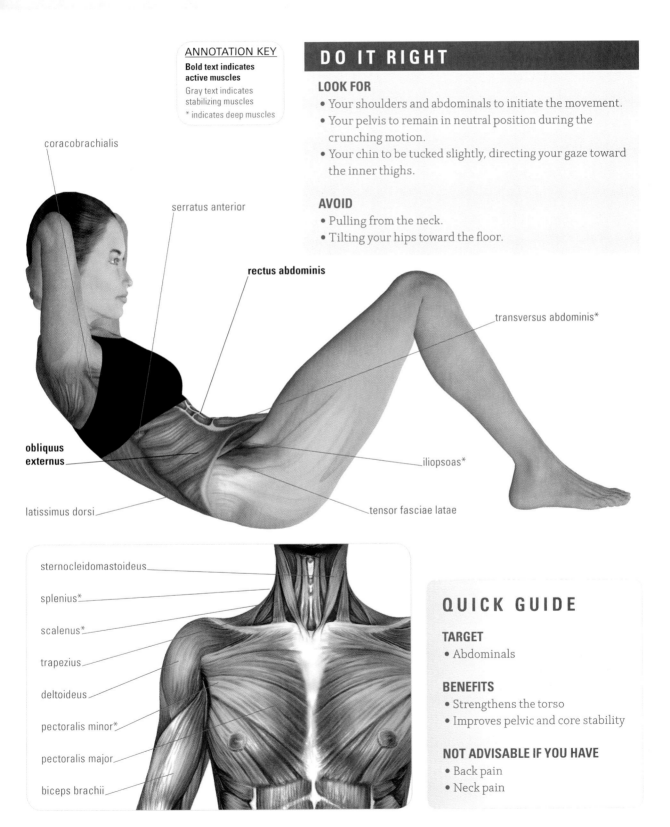

ANNOTATION KEY
Bold text indicates active muscles
Gray text indicates stabilizing muscles
* indicates deep muscles

coracobrachialis

serratus anterior

rectus abdominis

transversus abdominis*

obliquus externus

iliopsoas*

latissimus dorsi

tensor fasciae latae

sternocleidomastoideus

splenius*

scalenus*

trapezius

deltoideus

pectoralis minor*

pectoralis major

biceps brachii

DO IT RIGHT

LOOK FOR
- Your shoulders and abdominals to initiate the movement.
- Your pelvis to remain in neutral position during the crunching motion.
- Your chin to be tucked slightly, directing your gaze toward the inner thighs.

AVOID
- Pulling from the neck.
- Tilting your hips toward the floor.

QUICK GUIDE

TARGET
- Abdominals

BENEFITS
- Strengthens the torso
- Improves pelvic and core stability

NOT ADVISABLE IF YOU HAVE
- Back pain
- Neck pain

CROSSOVER CRUNCH

CORE STRENGTH

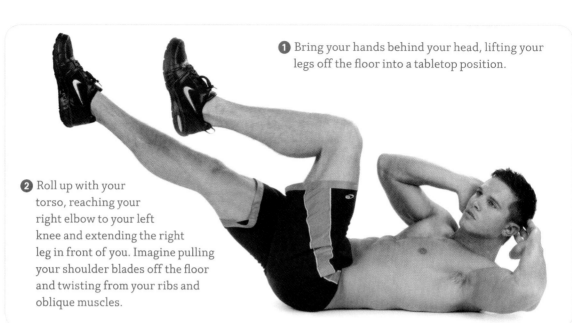

❶ Bring your hands behind your head, lifting your legs off the floor into a tabletop position.

❷ Roll up with your torso, reaching your right elbow to your left knee and extending the right leg in front of you. Imagine pulling your shoulder blades off the floor and twisting from your ribs and oblique muscles.

❸ Alternate sides. Repeat sequence six times.

QUICK GUIDE

TARGET
- Torso stability
- Abdominals

BENEFITS
- Stabilizes core
- Strengthens abdominals

NOT ADVISABLE IF YOU HAVE
- Neck issues
- Lower-back pain

BEST FOR

- rectus abdominis
- transversus abdominis
- obliquus externus
- obliquus internus
- rectus femoris
- vastus medialis
- sartorius
- tensor fasciae latae

MODIFICATION

Easier: Begin with both feet on the floor. Place the outside of one foot on top of your thigh near your knee. Reach your opposite elbow toward the knee of your raised leg. After six repetitions, repeat on the other side.

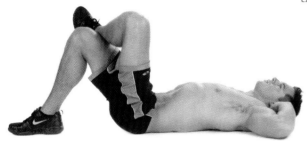

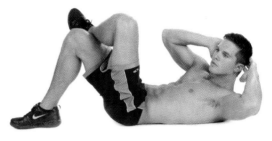

ANNOTATION KEY
Bold text indicates active muscles
Gray text indicates stabilizing muscles
* indicates deep muscles

DO IT RIGHT

LOOK FOR
- Your neck to remain long and your chin to remain away from your chest.
- Both hips to remain stable on the floor.

AVOID
- Pulling with your hands, bringing your chin toward your chest, or arching your back.
- Moving the active elbow faster than your shoulder.

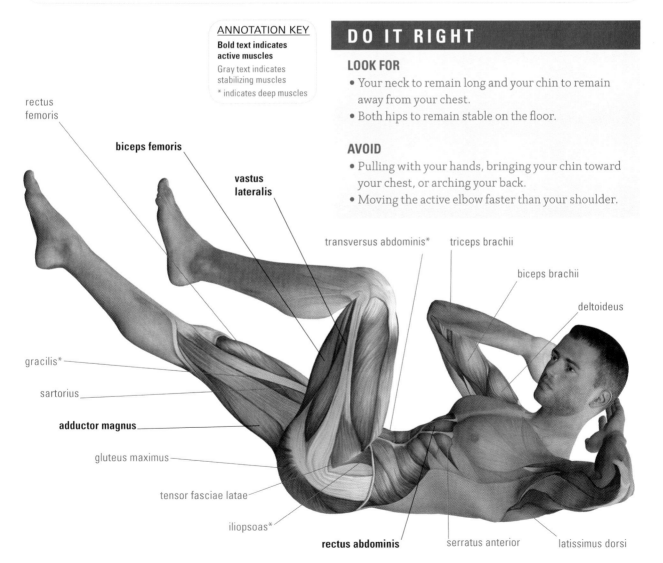

rectus femoris

biceps femoris

vastus lateralis

transversus abdominis*

triceps brachii

biceps brachii

deltoideus

gracilis*

sartorius

adductor magnus

gluteus maximus

tensor fasciae latae

iliopsoas*

rectus abdominis

serratus anterior

latissimus dorsi

LATERAL LOW LUNGE

CORE STRENGTH

1 Stand upright with your hips and arms outstretched in front of you, parallel to the floor.

DO IT RIGHT

LOOK FOR
- Your spine to remain neutral as you bend your hips.
- Your shoulders and neck to remain relaxed.
- Your knee to align with the toe of your bent leg.
- The gluteal muscles to be tight as you bend.

AVOID
- Craning your neck as you perform the movement.
- Lifting your feet off the floor.
- Arching or extending your back.

2 Step out to the left. Squat down on your right leg, bending at your hips, while maintaining a neutral spine. Begin to extend your left leg, keeping both feet flat on the floor.

3 Bend your right knee until your thigh is parallel to the floor, and your left leg is fully extended.

4 Keeping your arms parallel to the ground, squeeze your buttocks and press off your right leg to return to the starting position, and repeat. Repeat sequence ten times on each side.

QUICK GUIDE

TARGET
- Gluteal and thigh muscles

BENEFITS
- Strengthens the pelvic, trunk, and knee stabilizers

NOT ADVISABLE IF YOU HAVE
- Sharp knee pain
- Back pain
- Trouble bearing weight on one leg

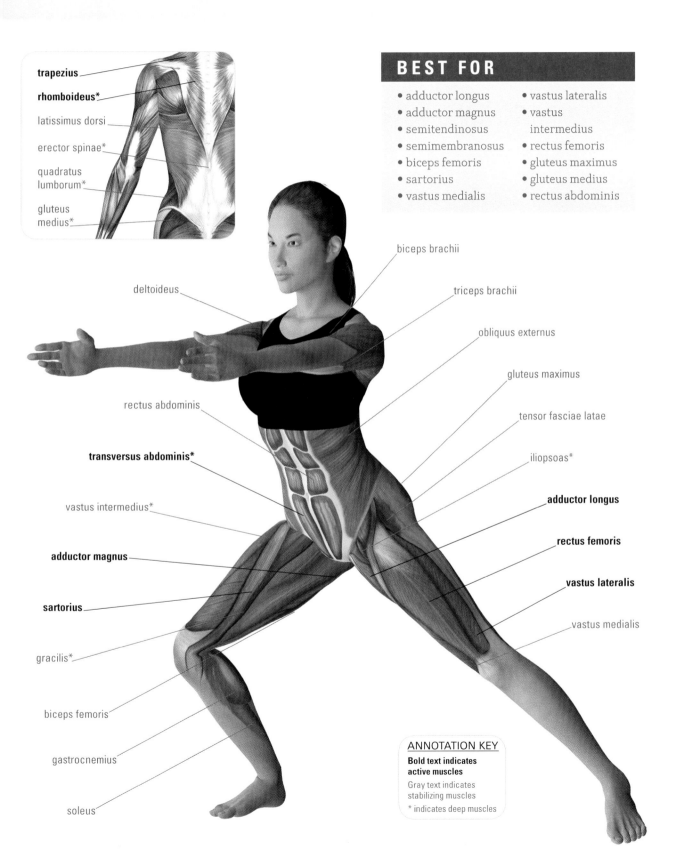

trapezius
rhomboideus*
latissimus dorsi
erector spinae*
quadratus lumborum*
gluteus medius*

BEST FOR

- adductor longus
- adductor magnus
- semitendinosus
- semimembranosus
- biceps femoris
- sartorius
- vastus medialis
- vastus lateralis
- vastus intermedius
- rectus femoris
- gluteus maximus
- gluteus medius
- rectus abdominis

biceps brachii

deltoideus

triceps brachii

obliquus externus

gluteus maximus

rectus abdominis

tensor fasciae latae

transversus abdominis*

iliopsoas*

adductor longus

vastus intermedius*

rectus femoris

adductor magnus

vastus lateralis

sartorius

vastus medialis

gracilis*

biceps femoris

gastrocnemius

soleus

ANNOTATION KEY
Bold text indicates active muscles
Gray text indicates stabilizing muscles
* indicates deep muscles

STEP-DOWN

1 Standing up straight on a firm step or block, plant your left foot firmly close to the edge, and allow the right foot to hang off the side. Flex the toes of your right foot.

DO IT RIGHT

LOOK FOR

- Your bent knee to align with your second toe—your knee should not rotate inward.
- Your knees and hips to move simultaneously as you bend.
- Your hips to remain behind your foot, leaning your torso forward as you lower into the bend.

AVOID

- Craning your neck.
- Placing weight on the foot being lowered to the floor—only allow a touch.

2 Lift your arms out in front of you for balance, keeping them parallel to the floor. Lower your torso as you bend at your hips and knees, dropping your right leg toward the floor.

3 Without rotating your torso or knee, press upward through your left leg to return to the starting position. Repeat fifteen times for two sets on each leg.

BEST FOR

- vastus medialis
- vastus lateralis
- vastus intermedius
- rectus femoris
- gluteus maximus
- gluteus medius
- semitendinosus
- semimembranosus
- biceps femoris

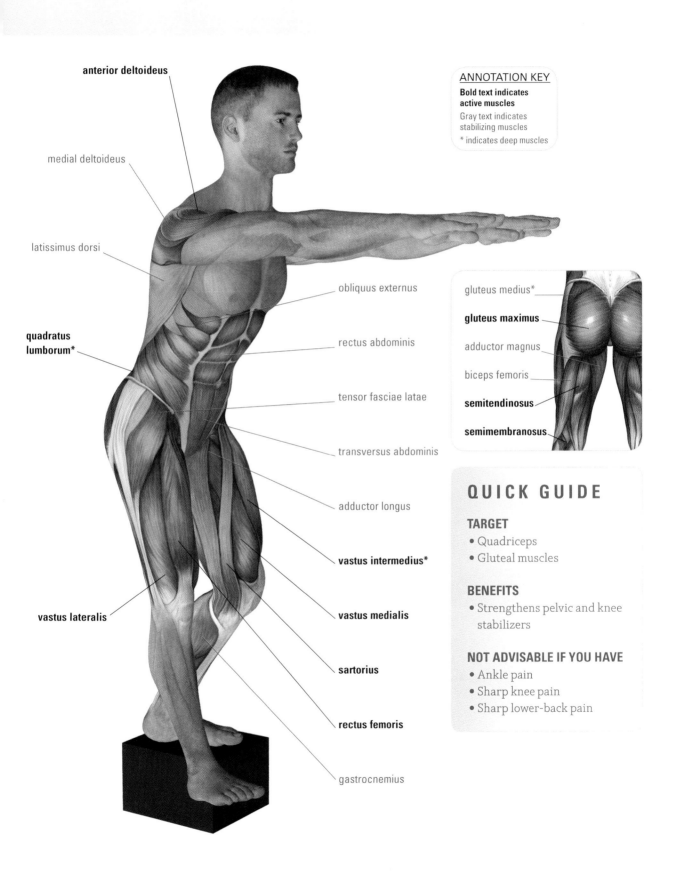

anterior deltoideus

medial deltoideus

latissimus dorsi

quadratus
lumborum*

vastus lateralis

obliquus externus

rectus abdominis

tensor fasciae latae

transversus abdominis

adductor longus

vastus intermedius*

vastus medialis

sartorius

rectus femoris

gastrocnemius

ANNOTATION KEY
Bold text indicates active muscles
Gray text indicates stabilizing muscles
* indicates deep muscles

gluteus medius*

gluteus maximus

adductor magnus

biceps femoris

semitendinosus

semimembranosus

QUICK GUIDE

TARGET
- Quadriceps
- Gluteal muscles

BENEFITS
- Strengthens pelvic and knee stabilizers

NOT ADVISABLE IF YOU HAVE
- Ankle pain
- Sharp knee pain
- Sharp lower-back pain

TENDON STRETCH

CORE STRENGTH

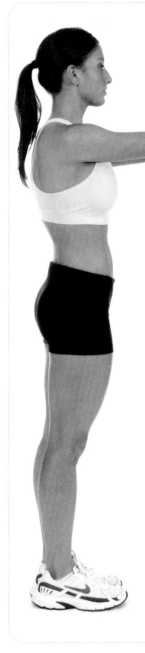

1 Standing with your feet together and parallel, extend your arms in front of your body for stability.

With your feet planted firmly on the floor, curl your toes upward.

DO IT RIGHT

LOOK FOR
- Your chest to remain upright.
- Your abdominals to be pulled in toward your spine.
- Your toes to curl upward throughout the movement.

AVOID
- Allowing your heels to come off the floor.
- Rising to the standing position too quickly.

2 Draw in your abdominal muscles, and bend into a squat. Keep your heels planted on the floor and your chest as upright as possible, resisting the urge to bend too far forward.

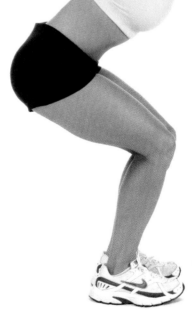

3 Exhale, returning to the original position. Imagine pressing into the floor as you rise, creating your body's own resistance in your leg muscles. Repeat five to six times.

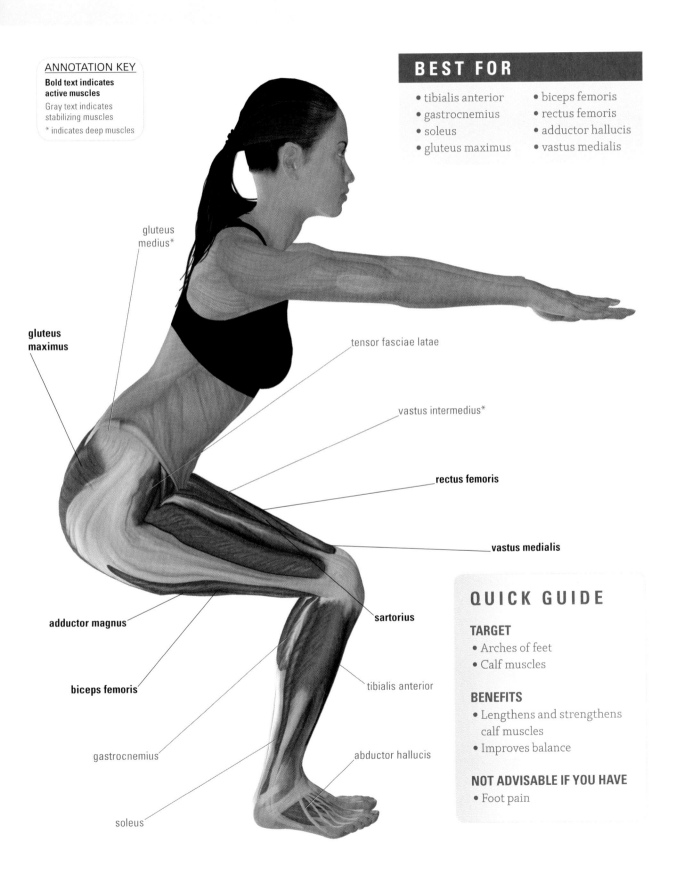

ANNOTATION KEY

Bold text indicates active muscles

Gray text indicates stabilizing muscles

* indicates deep muscles

BEST FOR

- tibialis anterior
- gastrocnemius
- soleus
- gluteus maximus
- biceps femoris
- rectus femoris
- adductor hallucis
- vastus medialis

gluteus medius*

gluteus maximus

tensor fasciae latae

vastus intermedius*

rectus femoris

vastus medialis

adductor magnus

sartorius

biceps femoris

tibialis anterior

gastrocnemius

abductor hallucis

soleus

QUICK GUIDE

TARGET
- Arches of feet
- Calf muscles

BENEFITS
- Lengthens and strengthens calf muscles
- Improves balance

NOT ADVISABLE IF YOU HAVE
- Foot pain

ABDOMINAL KICK

CORE STRENGTH

1 Pull your right knee toward your chest and straighten your left leg, raising it about 45 degrees from the floor.

2 Place your right hand on your right ankle, and your left hand on your right knee (this maintains proper alignment of leg).

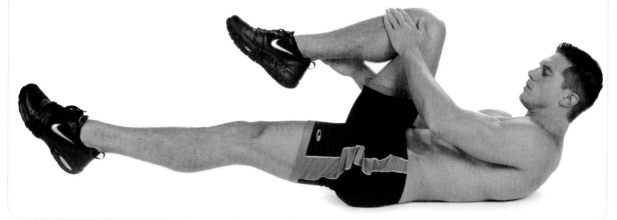

3 Switch your legs two times, switching your hand placement simultaneously.

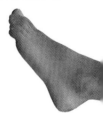

QUICK GUIDE

TARGET
• Torso stability
• Abdominals

BENEFITS
• Stabilizes core while extremities are in motion
• Strengthens abdominals

NOT ADVISABLE IF YOU HAVE
• Neck issues
• Lower-back pain

DO IT RIGHT

LOOK FOR
• Your outside hand to be placed on the ankle of your bent leg, and your inside hand to be placed on your bent knee.
• The top of your sternum to be lifted forward.

AVOID
• Allowing your lower back to rise up off the floor; use your abdominals to stabilize core while switching legs.

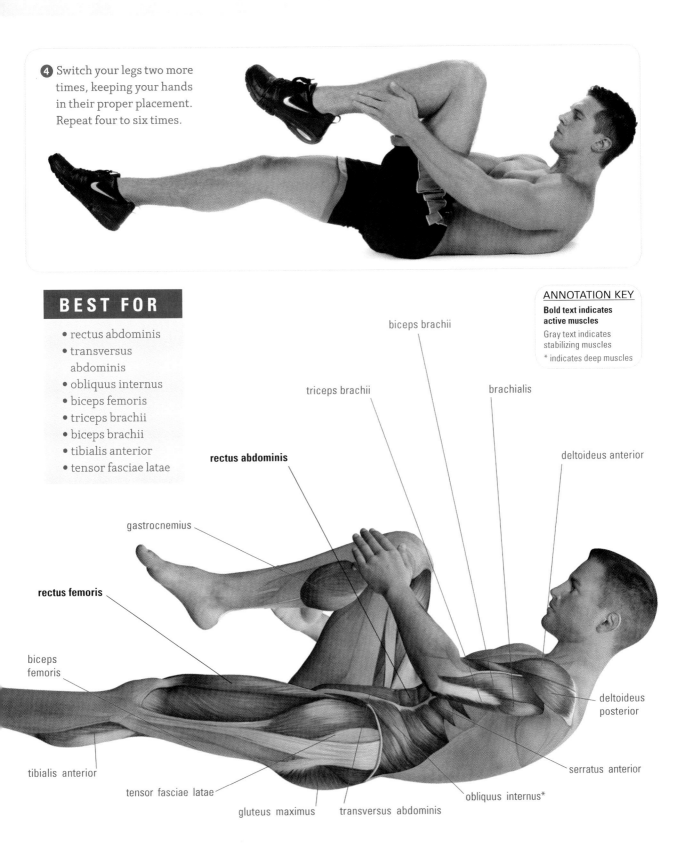

4 Switch your legs two more times, keeping your hands in their proper placement. Repeat four to six times.

BEST FOR

- rectus abdominis
- transversus abdominis
- obliquus internus
- biceps femoris
- triceps brachii
- biceps brachii
- tibialis anterior
- tensor fasciae latae

ANNOTATION KEY
Bold text indicates active muscles
Gray text indicates stabilizing muscles
* indicates deep muscles

biceps brachii

triceps brachii

brachialis

deltoideus anterior

rectus abdominis

gastrocnemius

rectus femoris

biceps femoris

deltoideus posterior

tibialis anterior

tensor fasciae latae

gluteus maximus

transversus abdominis

obliquus internus*

serratus anterior

POWER SQUAT

CORE STRENGTH

1 Stand straight, holding a weighted ball in front of your torso.

2 Shift your weight to your left foot, and bend your right knee, lifting your right foot toward your buttocks. Bend your elbows and draw the ball toward the outside of your right ear.

DO IT RIGHT

LOOK FOR
- The ball to create an arc in the air.
- Your hips and knees to be aligned throughout the movement.
- Your shoulders and neck to remain relaxed.

AVOID
- Allowing your knee to extend beyond your toes as you bend and rotate.
- Moving your foot from its starting position.
- Flexing your spine.

3 Maintaining a neutral spine, bend at your hips and knee. Lower your torso toward your left side, bringing the ball toward your right ankle.

4 Press into your left leg and straighten your knee and torso, returning to the starting position. Repeat fifteen times for two sets on each leg.

QUICK GUIDE

TARGET
- Stabilizers of the body
- Gluteal and thigh strength

BENEFITS
- Improves balance
- Improves pelvic, trunk, and knee stabilization
- Promotes stronger movement patterns

NOT ADVISABLE IF YOU HAVE
- Sharp knee pain
- Lower-back pain
- Shoulder pain

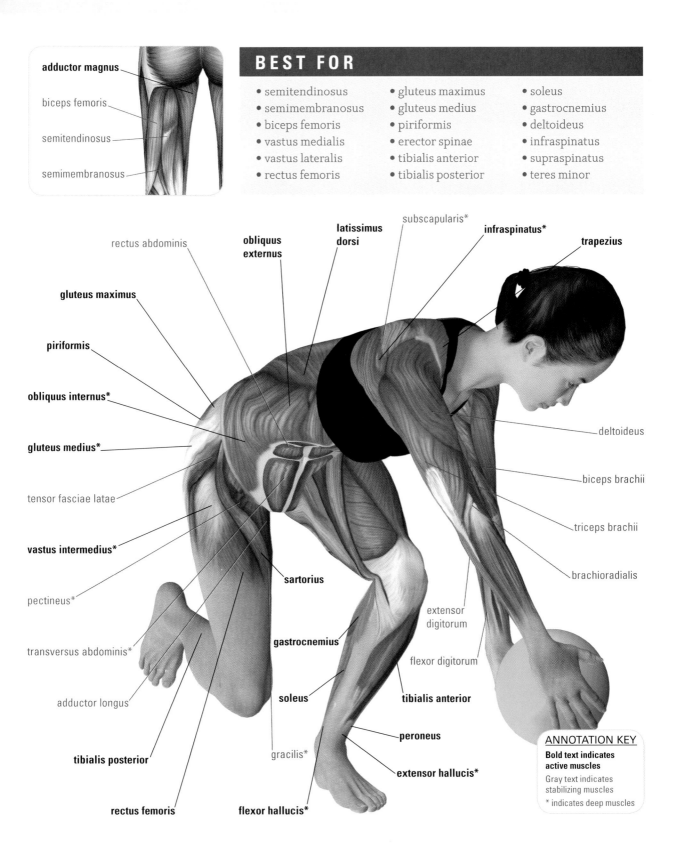

adductor magnus

biceps femoris

semitendinosus

semimembranosus

BEST FOR

- semitendinosus
- semimembranosus
- biceps femoris
- vastus medialis
- vastus lateralis
- rectus femoris

- gluteus maximus
- gluteus medius
- piriformis
- erector spinae
- tibialis anterior
- tibialis posterior

- soleus
- gastrocnemius
- deltoideus
- infraspinatus
- supraspinatus
- teres minor

rectus abdominis

obliquus externus

latissimus dorsi

subscapularis*

infraspinatus*

trapezius

gluteus maximus

piriformis

obliquus internus*

gluteus medius*

tensor fasciae latae

vastus intermedius*

pectineus*

transversus abdominis*

adductor longus

tibialis posterior

rectus femoris

sartorius

gastrocnemius

soleus

gracilis*

flexor hallucis*

deltoideus

biceps brachii

triceps brachii

brachioradialis

extensor digitorum

flexor digitorum

tibialis anterior

peroneus

extensor hallucis*

ANNOTATION KEY

Bold text indicates active muscles

Gray text indicates stabilizing muscles

* indicates deep muscles

LEMON SQUEEZER

CORE STRENGTH

1 Lie supine on the floor. Lift your legs, head, neck, and shoulders slightly off the floor, being careful not to arch your lower back. Your arms should be raised and parallel to the floor.

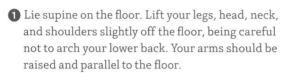

BEST FOR

- rectus abdominis
- obliquus internus
- obliquus externus
- transversus abdominis
- tensor fasciae latae
- vastus intermedius
- rectus femoris
- vastus medialis
- iliacus
- piriformis
- iliacus

2 Pulling your knees in toward your chest, reach your arms forward to your ankles, so that your torso lifts completely off the floor.

3 Slowly open up, lengthening your legs and lowering your torso back to the starting position.

4 Repeat the motion without completely lying down on the mat. Repeat fifteen times for two sets.

QUICK GUIDE

TARGET
• Abdominals

BENEFITS
• Increases abdominal endurance
• Strengthens hip flexors

NOT ADVISABLE IF YOU HAVE
• Lower-back pain

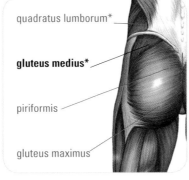

quadratus lumborum*
gluteus medius*
piriformis
gluteus maximus

ANNOTATION KEY
Bold text indicates active muscles
Gray text indicates stabilizing muscles
* indicates deep muscles

rectus abdominis

obliquus externus

obliquus internus*

vastus lateralis

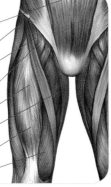

transversus abdominis*
tensor fasciae latae
iliopsoas*
iliacus*
vastus intermedius*
adductor longus
rectus femoris
vastus medialis

DO IT RIGHT

LOOK FOR
• The chin to remain tucked.
• Your thigh muscles to be firm throughout the exercise.

AVOID
• Allowing your shoulders to lift up toward your ears.

V-UP

1 Lie on your back with your legs raised at an angle between 45 and 90 degrees.

BEST FOR

- rectus abdominis
- tensor fasciae latae
- rectus femoris
- vastus lateralis
- vastus medialis
- vastus intermedius
- adductor longus
- pectineus
- brachialis

2 Inhale, reaching your arms toward the ceiling as you lift your head and shoulders off the floor.

3 Exhale, and, while rolling through the spine, lift your rib cage off the floor to just before the sit bones.

QUICK GUIDE

TARGET
- Abdominals

BENEFITS
- Strengthens the abdominals while mobilizing the spine

NOT ADVISABLE IF YOU HAVE
- Advanced osteoporosis
- A herniated disk
- Lower-back pain

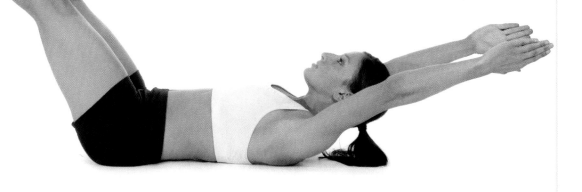

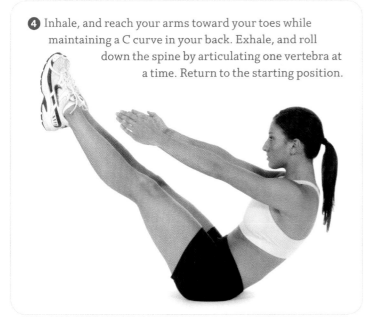

④ Inhale, and reach your arms toward your toes while maintaining a C curve in your back. Exhale, and roll down the spine by articulating one vertebra at a time. Return to the starting position.

DO IT RIGHT

LOOK FOR
- Articulation through the spine on the way up and on the way down.
- Your neck to remain elongated and relaxed, minimizing the tension in your upper spine.

AVOID
- Using momentum to carry you through the exercise. Use your abdominal muscles to lift your legs and torso.

ANNOTATION KEY
Bold text indicates active muscles
Gray text indicates stabilizing muscles
* indicates deep muscles

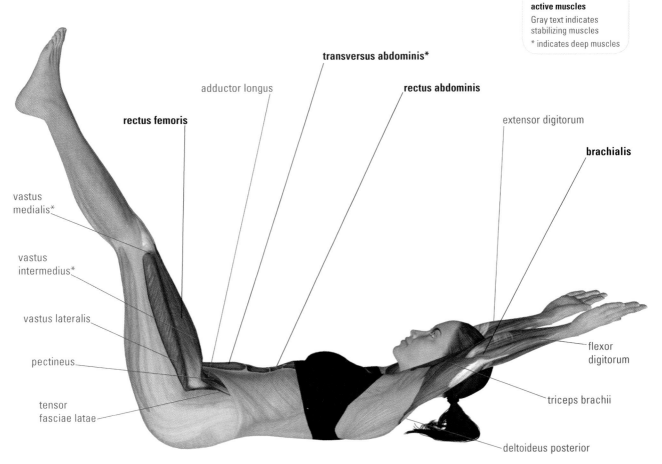

transversus abdominis*

adductor longus

rectus abdominis

rectus femoris

extensor digitorum

brachialis

vastus medialis*

vastus intermedius*

vastus lateralis

pectineus

tensor fasciae latae

flexor digitorum

triceps brachii

deltoideus posterior

RUSSIAN TWIST

CORE STRENGTH

BEST FOR

- rectus abdominis
- obliquus internus
- obliquus externus
- transversus abdominis
- vastus intermedius
- rectus femoris
- iliacus
- iliopsoas

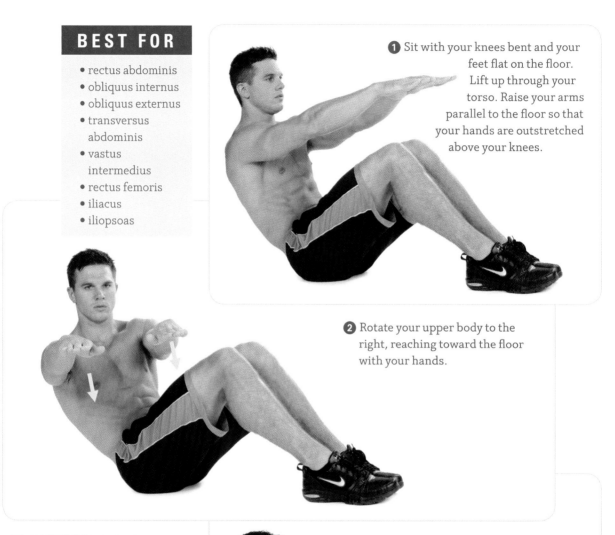

1 Sit with your knees bent and your feet flat on the floor. Lift up through your torso. Raise your arms parallel to the floor so that your hands are outstretched above your knees.

2 Rotate your upper body to the right, reaching toward the floor with your hands.

3 Pass through the center and rotate to the left. Repeat ten times on each side.

QUICK GUIDE

TARGET
- Abdominals
- Hip flexors
- Quadriceps

BENEFITS
- Increases abdominal endurance
- Strengthens hip flexors

MODIFICATION
More difficult: Lift your feet off the floor, and rotate your torso from side to side, pulling your knees in and out as you twist.

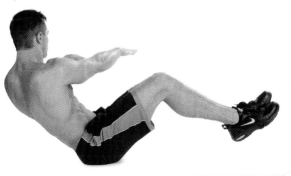

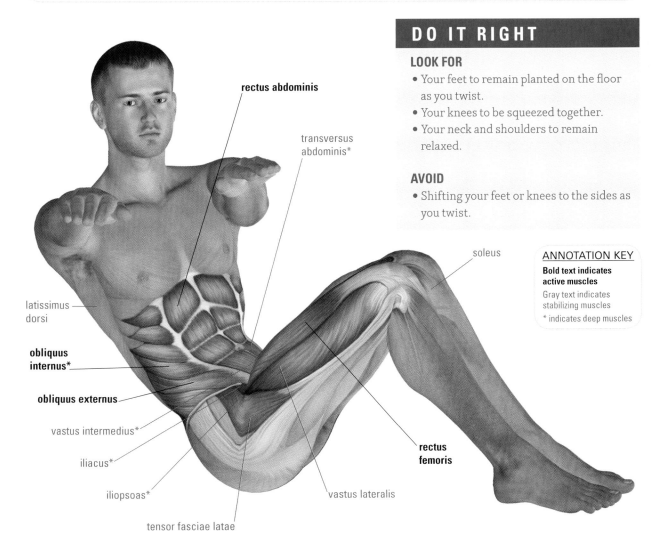

rectus abdominis

transversus abdominis*

latissimus dorsi

obliquus internus*

obliquus externus

vastus intermedius*

iliacus*

iliopsoas*

tensor fasciae latae

vastus lateralis

rectus femoris

soleus

DO IT RIGHT

LOOK FOR
• Your feet to remain planted on the floor as you twist.
• Your knees to be squeezed together.
• Your neck and shoulders to remain relaxed.

AVOID
• Shifting your feet or knees to the sides as you twist.

ANNOTATION KEY
Bold text indicates active muscles
Gray text indicates stabilizing muscles
* indicates deep muscles

PLANK KNEE PULL-IN

CORE STRENGTH

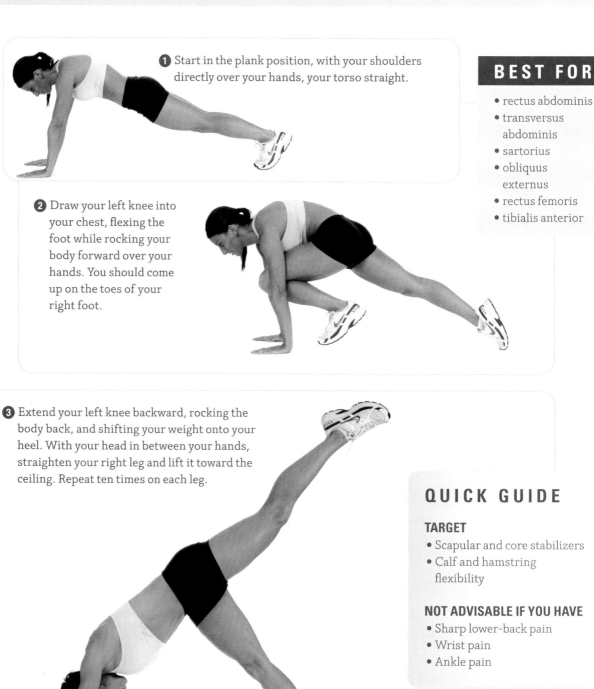

❶ Start in the plank position, with your shoulders directly over your hands, your torso straight.

❷ Draw your left knee into your chest, flexing the foot while rocking your body forward over your hands. You should come up on the toes of your right foot.

❸ Extend your left knee backward, rocking the body back, and shifting your weight onto your heel. With your head in between your hands, straighten your right leg and lift it toward the ceiling. Repeat ten times on each leg.

BEST FOR

- rectus abdominis
- transversus abdominis
- sartorius
- obliquus externus
- rectus femoris
- tibialis anterior

QUICK GUIDE

TARGET
- Scapular and core stabilizers
- Calf and hamstring flexibility

NOT ADVISABLE IF YOU HAVE
- Sharp lower-back pain
- Wrist pain
- Ankle pain

DO IT RIGHT

LOOK FOR
• Your shoulders to align over your hands and your toes to flex during the inward movement.

AVOID
• Bending the knee of the supporting leg.

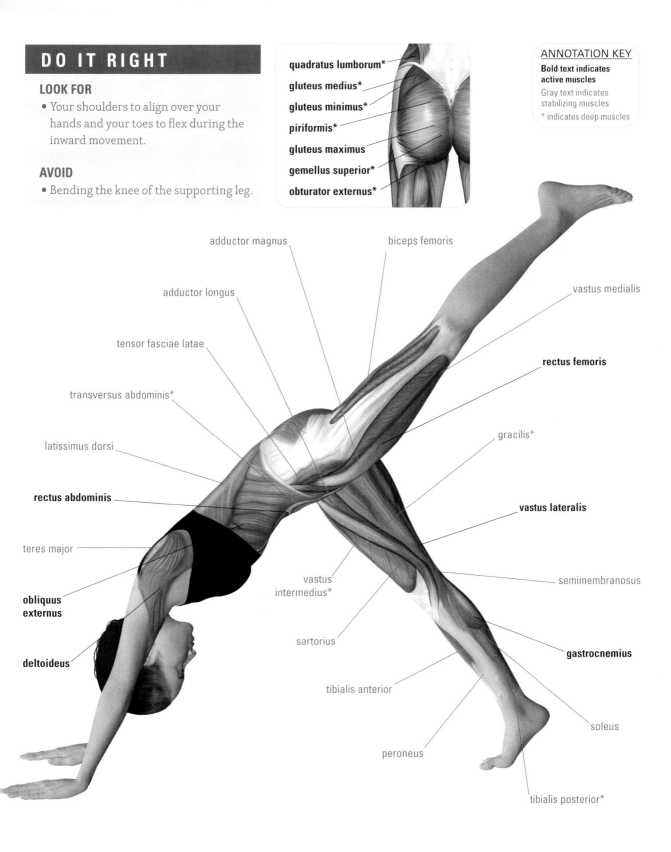

quadratus lumborum*

gluteus medius*

gluteus minimus*

piriformis*

gluteus maximus

gemellus superior*

obturator externus*

adductor magnus

biceps femoris

vastus medialis

adductor longus

rectus femoris

tensor fasciae latae

transversus abdominis*

gracilis*

latissimus dorsi

vastus lateralis

rectus abdominis

teres major

semimembranosus

obliquus externus

vastus intermedius*

deltoideus

sartorius

gastrocnemius

tibialis anterior

soleus

peroneus

tibialis posterior*

SIDE-LIFT BEND

CORE STRENGTH

1 Lie on your left side with your right arm placed behind your head and your left arm lying flat on top of your thigh. Tightly press your legs together.

2 Tighten your abdominals and lift both legs off the floor.

QUICK GUIDE

TARGET
- Obliques
- Abdominals

BENEFITS
- Strengthens and stabilizes the body

NOT ADVISABLE IF YOU HAVE
- Lower-back pain

BEST FOR

- rectus abdominis
- transversus abdominis
- obliquus externus
- obliquus internus

vastus medialis

sartorius

vastus lateralis

ANNOTATION KEY
Bold text indicates active muscles
Gray text indicates stabilizing muscles
* indicates deep muscles

DO IT RIGHT

LOOK FOR

- Your buttocks to be squeezed before lifting to better stabilize the pelvis.
- Your neck to be elongated.
- Your hand to slide down on the top leg as you crunch up.

3 Sliding your right hand down your outstretched leg, lift your head, and crunch your oblique muscles from your upper body and lower body simultaneously. Repeat ten times on each side.

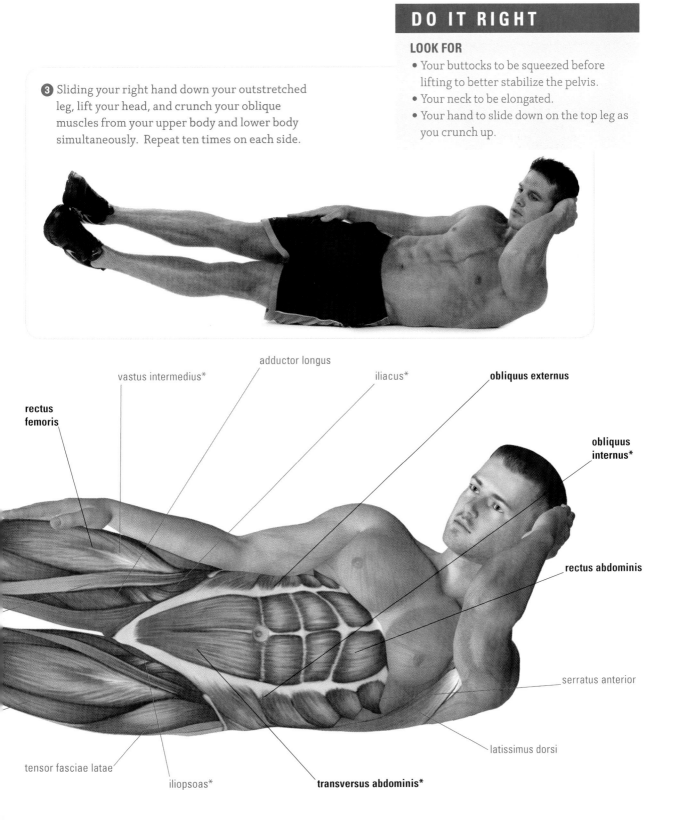

rectus
femoris

vastus intermedius*

adductor longus

iliacus*

obliquus externus

obliquus internus*

rectus abdominis

serratus anterior

latissimus dorsi

tensor fasciae latae

iliopsoas*

transversus abdominis*

THE TWIST

QUICK GUIDE

TARGET
- Shoulders
- Abdominals

BENEFITS
- Provides a total-body workout
- Builds endurance

NOT ADVISABLE IF YOU HAVE
- Shoulder issues
- Back pain
- Wrist injury

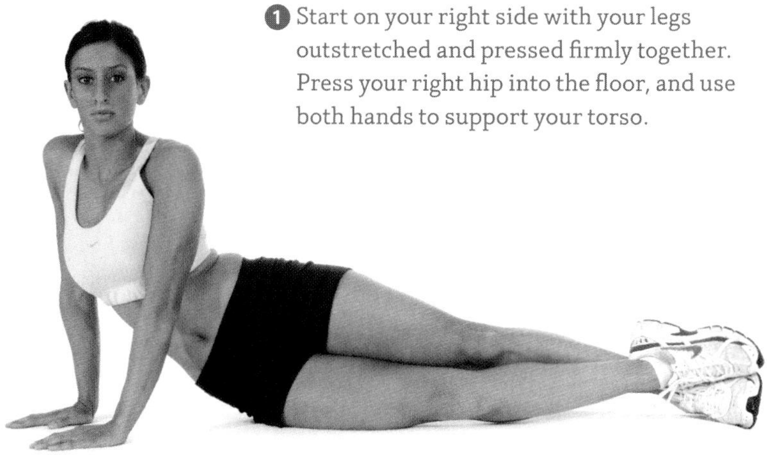

❶ Start on your right side with your legs outstretched and pressed firmly together. Press your right hip into the floor, and use both hands to support your torso.

❷ Position your right hand directly beneath your shoulder and press your body up into a side plank with side-arm balance.

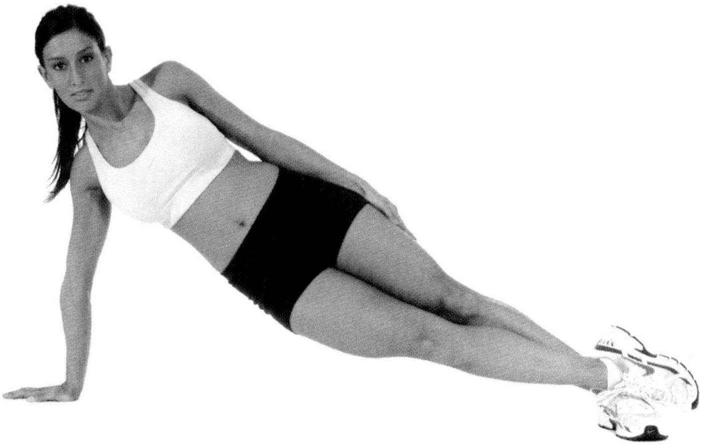

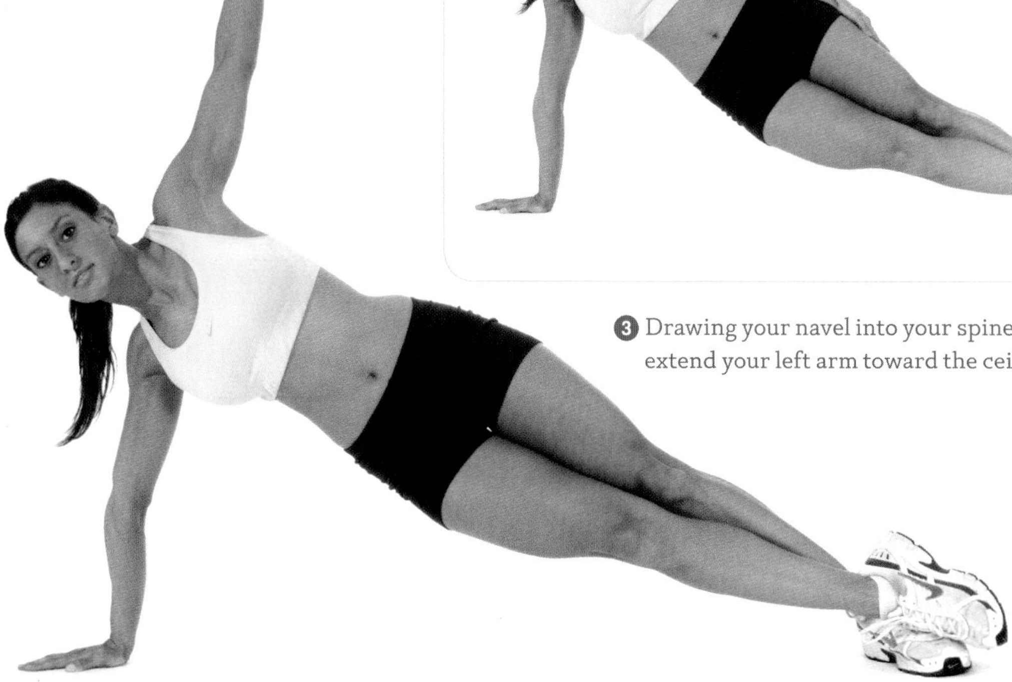

❸ Drawing your navel into your spine, extend your left arm toward the ceiling.

DO IT RIGHT

LOOK FOR

- Your limbs to be elongated as much as possible.
- Your shoulders to remain stable.
- Your hips to be lifted up high to reduce the weight on your upper body.

AVOID

- Allowing your shoulder to sink into its socket.

BEST FOR

- latissimus dorsi
- rectus abdominis
- obliquus internus
- obliquus externus
- transversus abdominis
- adductor magnus
- adductor longus
- deltoideus

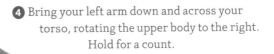

4 Bring your left arm down and across your torso, rotating the upper body to the right. Hold for a count.

5 Return to the starting position, with your hip on the floor and both hands supporting your torso. Repeat sequence four to six times, and then switch sides.

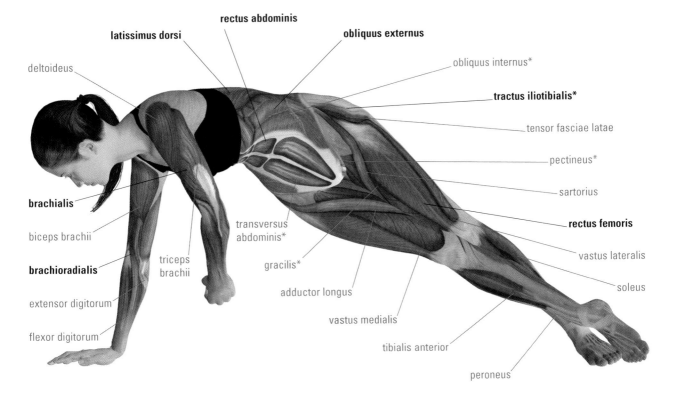

- latissimus dorsi
- rectus abdominis
- obliquus externus
- obliquus internus*
- deltoideus
- tractus iliotibialis*
- tensor fasciae latae
- pectineus*
- sartorius
- rectus femoris
- vastus lateralis
- soleus
- brachialis
- biceps brachii
- brachioradialis
- triceps brachii
- transversus abdominis*
- gracilis*
- adductor longus
- vastus medialis
- tibialis anterior
- peroneus
- extensor digitorum
- flexor digitorum

HIP TWIST

CORE STRENGTH

BEST FOR

- tensor fasciae latae
- rectus femoris
- vastus lateralis
- biceps femoris
- gluteus maximus
- gluteus medius
- iliotibial band
- sartorius
- vastus medialis
- vastus intermedius
- adductor longus

1 Begin by sitting on the floor with your arms behind your body, supporting your weight. Your legs should be parallel and raised to a high diagonal.

2 Engage your abdominals and shoulders for stabilization.

3 Start to bring both legs across the body to the right.

4 Continue to circle your legs across your body and down as low as pelvic stabilization can be maintained.

5 Return your legs to the starting position. Repeat two to six times in each direction.

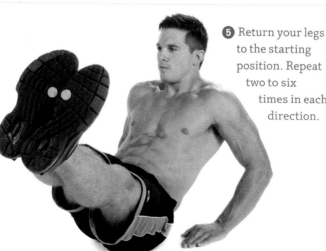

DO IT RIGHT

LOOK FOR
- Your legs to be lengthened as you move from side to side.
- Your arms to push out of your shoulders to better engage your torso.
- Your neck to be elongated.

AVOID
- Tensing your neck and shoulder muscles.

QUICK GUIDE

TARGET
• Abdominals

BENEFITS
• Strengthens abdominals against gravity and weight of legs

NOT ADVISABLE IF YOU HAVE
• Back pain
• Hip instability

ANNOTATION KEY
Bold text indicates active muscles
Gray text indicates stabilizing muscles
* indicates deep muscles

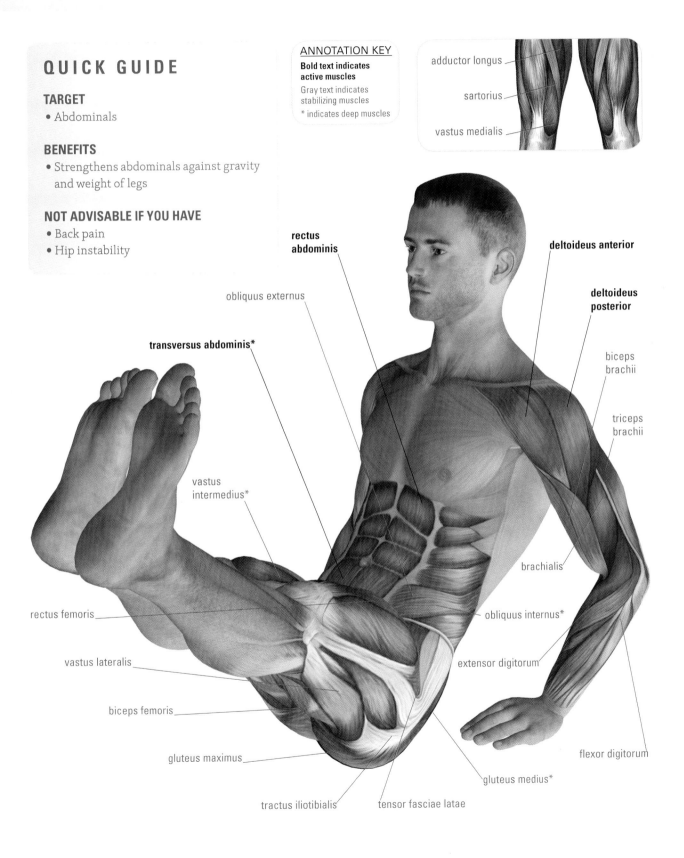

adductor longus
sartorius
vastus medialis

rectus abdominis

obliquus externus

transversus abdominis*

deltoideus anterior

deltoideus posterior

biceps brachii

triceps brachii

vastus intermedius*

brachialis

rectus femoris

obliquus internus*

vastus lateralis

extensor digitorum

biceps femoris

gluteus maximus

flexor digitorum

tractus iliotibialis

tensor fasciae latae

gluteus medius*

KNEELING SIDE LIFT

CORE STRENGTH

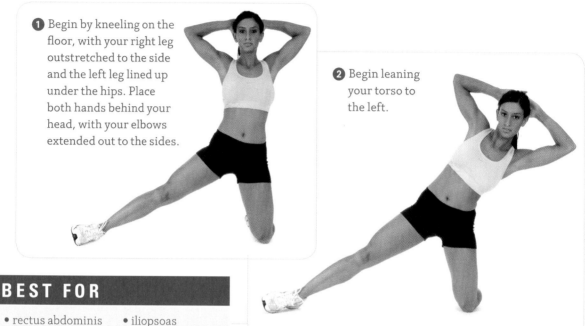

1 Begin by kneeling on the floor, with your right leg outstretched to the side and the left leg lined up under the hips. Place both hands behind your head, with your elbows extended out to the sides.

2 Begin leaning your torso to the left.

BEST FOR

- rectus abdominis
- transversus abdominis
- obliquus externus
- adductor longus
- iliopsoas
- iliacus
- gracilis
- biceps femoris
- vastus lateralis

3 Lift your right leg up off the floor, bringing it as high as your hips. Repeat sequence five to six times. Switch sides, and repeat the sequence with your left leg.

QUICK GUIDE

TARGET
- Abductor muscles
- Abdominals
- Gluteal muscles

BENEFITS
- Trims the waistline

NOT ADVISABLE IF YOU HAVE
- Knee pain or injury
- Back pain

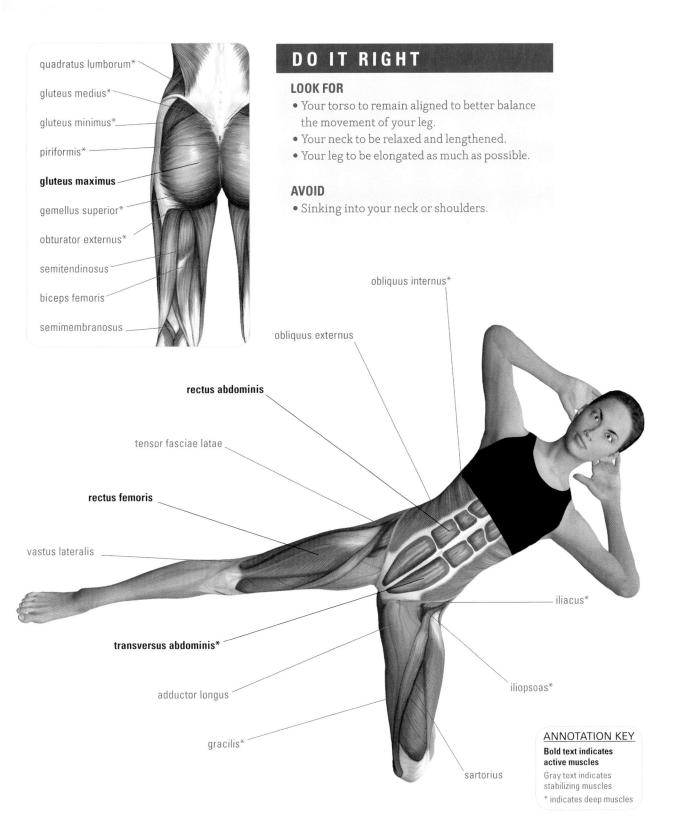

quadratus lumborum*

gluteus medius*

gluteus minimus*

piriformis*

gluteus maximus

gemellus superior*

obturator externus*

semitendinosus

biceps femoris

semimembranosus

DO IT RIGHT

LOOK FOR
- Your torso to remain aligned to better balance the movement of your leg.
- Your neck to be relaxed and lengthened.
- Your leg to be elongated as much as possible.

AVOID
- Sinking into your neck or shoulders.

obliquus internus*

obliquus externus

rectus abdominis

tensor fasciae latae

rectus femoris

vastus lateralis

transversus abdominis*

adductor longus

gracilis*

iliacus*

iliopsoas*

sartorius

ANNOTATION KEY
Bold text indicates active muscles

Gray text indicates stabilizing muscles

* indicates deep muscles

KNEELING SIDE KICK

CORE STRENGTH

BEST FOR

- rectus abdominis
- transversus abdominis
- obliquus externus
- obliquus internus
- gluteus medius
- gluteus maximus
- adductor longus
- gracilis
- tensor fasciae latae
- sartorius
- rectus femoris
- iliacus
- iliopsoas
- vastus lateralis

1 Kneel with your right hand on the floor directly below your shoulder, with the fingers pointing outward. Place your left hand behind your head.

2 Lift your left leg to the height of your hip and straighten it, reaching out of your heel. Keep your whole body aligned in one plane so that there is no rotation.

3 Kick your left leg straight out in front of you, flexing your foot and trying not to move at your waist.

QUICK GUIDE

TARGET
- Leg abductors
- Abdominals

NOT ADVISABLE IF YOU HAVE
- Wrist issues
- Severe back pain
- Shoulder issues

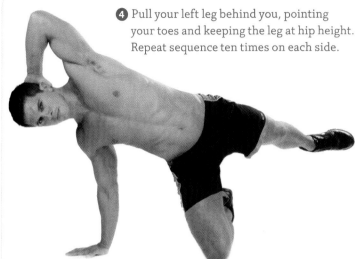

4 Pull your left leg behind you, pointing your toes and keeping the leg at hip height. Repeat sequence ten times on each side.

DO IT RIGHT

LOOK FOR
- Your weight to bear on the palm of your hand to help maintain balance.
- Your neck to remain long and relaxed.
- Your body to align so that your shoulders, hips, and legs line up to better activate deep muscles.

AVOID
- Wobbling with movement of the leg—instead, make the movement smaller.

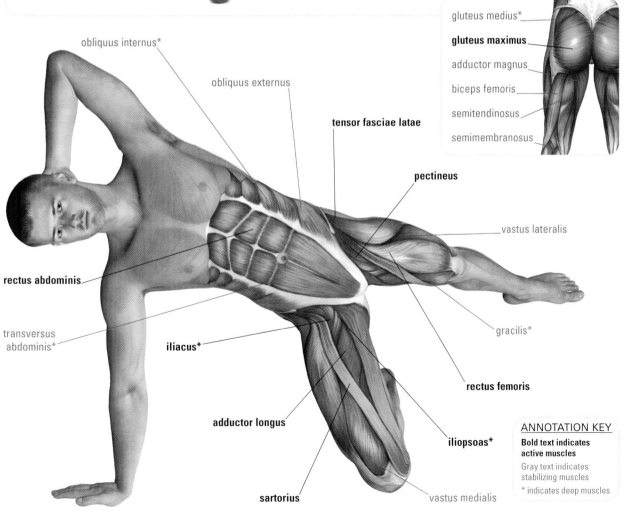

obliquus internus*

obliquus externus

tensor fasciae latae

gluteus medius*

gluteus maximus

adductor magnus

biceps femoris

semitendinosus

semimembranosus

pectineus

vastus lateralis

rectus abdominis

transversus abdominis*

iliacus*

gracilis*

rectus femoris

adductor longus

iliopsoas*

sartorius

vastus medialis

ANNOTATION KEY
Bold text indicates active muscles

Gray text indicates stabilizing muscles

* indicates deep muscles

ABDOMINAL HIP LIFT

QUICK GUIDE

TARGET
- Abdominals
- Triceps

BENEFITS
- Strengthens core and pelvic stabilizers
- Firms and tones lower abdominals

NOT ADVISABLE IF YOU HAVE
- Back pain
- Neck pain
- Shoulder pain

1 Lie down with your legs in the air and crossed at the ankles, knees straight. Place your arms on the floor, straight by your sides.

2 Pinching your legs together and squeezing your buttocks, press into the back of your arms to lift your hips upward.

3 Slowly return your hips to the floor. Repeat ten times, then switch with the opposite leg crossed in the front.

DO IT RIGHT

LOOK FOR
- Your legs to remain straight and firm throughout the exercise.
- Your neck and shoulders to be relaxed as you lift the hips.

AVOID
- Jerking your movements or using momentum to lift the hips.

BEST FOR

- rectus abdominis
- transversus abdominis
- vastus intermedius
- tensor fasciae latae
- gluteus maximus
- gluteus medius
- triceps brachii
- rectus femoris
- iliacus
- iliopsoas

quadratus lumborum*

gluteus medius*

piriformis*

gluteus maximus

MODIFICATION

More difficult: Keeping your hips on the floor, raise your arms toward the ceiling. Reach toward your toes as you lift your shoulders off the floor.

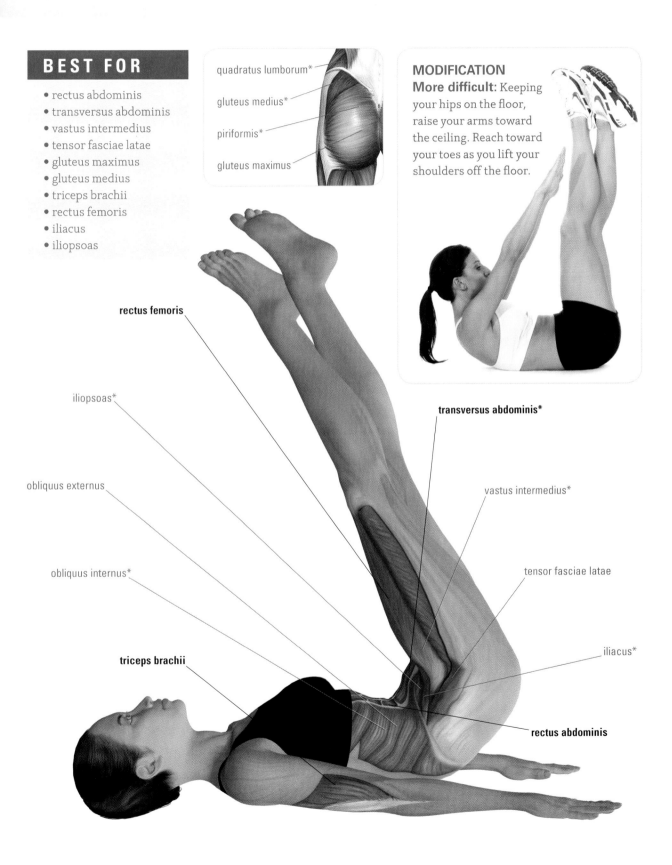

rectus femoris

iliopsoas*

obliquus externus

obliquus internus*

triceps brachii

transversus abdominis*

vastus intermedius*

tensor fasciae latae

iliacus*

rectus abdominis

HAND WALK-OUT

CORE STRENGTH

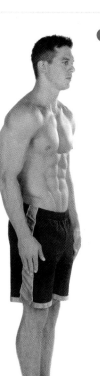

1 Stand straight, arms at your sides.

2 Bend forward from the waist, and place your hands on the floor in front of you, at a distance slightly wider than your feet. Keep your knees as straight as possible.

3 Shift your weight to your hands, and slowly "walk" them forward, while keeping the knees straight, the hips up, and the spine straight.

4 Return by walking back toward the starting position and pushing your hips upward, folding the torso at the hips.

DO IT RIGHT

LOOK FOR
- Your spine and legs to remain straight.
- A controlled, steady movement.

AVOID
- Bending your knees.
- Allowing your spine to sag in the middle.
- Bending your elbows.

QUICK GUIDE

TARGET
- Torso stability
- Abdominals

BENEFITS
- Stabilizes core
- Strengthens abdominals

NOT ADVISABLE IF YOU HAVE
- Shoulder issues
- Lower-back pain

BEST FOR

- pectoralis major
- pectoralis minor
- coracobrachialis
- deltoideus anterior
- triceps brachii
- iliopsoas
- vastus lateralis
- vastus medialis
- vastus intermedius
- rectus femoris
- transversus abdominis
- serratus anterior
- erector spinae
- trapezius
- latissimus dorsi
- quadratus lumborum
- brachialis
- tibialis anterior
- flexor carpi radialis
- extensor digitorum
- extensor carpi radialis
- biceps brachii

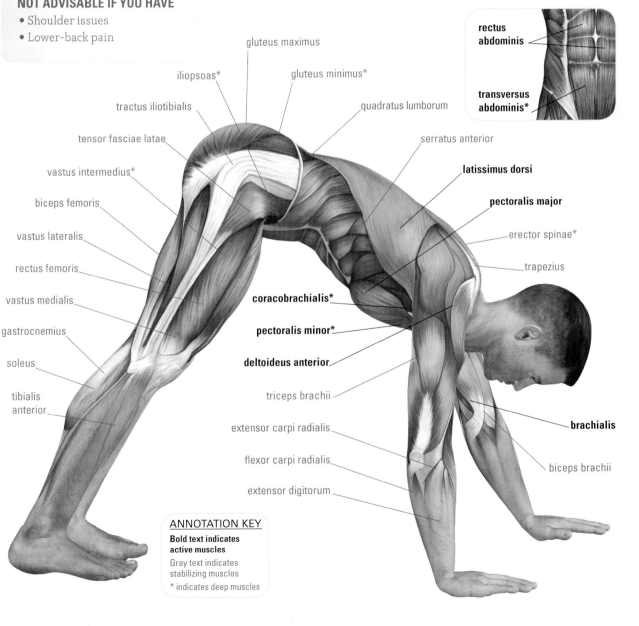

gluteus maximus

iliopsoas*

gluteus minimus*

tractus iliotibialis

quadratus lumborum

tensor fasciae latae

serratus anterior

vastus intermedius*

latissimus dorsi

biceps femoris

pectoralis major

vastus lateralis

erector spinae*

rectus femoris

trapezius

vastus medialis

coracobrachialis*

gastrocnemius

pectoralis minor*

soleus

deltoideus anterior

tibialis anterior

triceps brachii

brachialis

extensor carpi radialis

flexor carpi radialis

biceps brachii

extensor digitorum

rectus abdominis

transversus abdominis*

ANNOTATION KEY
Bold text indicates active muscles
Gray text indicates stabilizing muscles
* indicates deep muscles

CHAIR ABDOMINAL CRUNCH

CORE STRENGTH

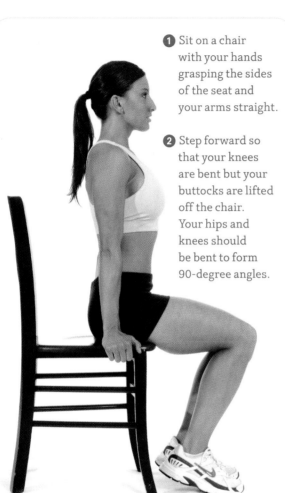

1 Sit on a chair with your hands grasping the sides of the seat and your arms straight.

2 Step forward so that your knees are bent but your buttocks are lifted off the chair. Your hips and knees should be bent to form 90-degree angles.

DO IT RIGHT

LOOK FOR
- Your spine to be neutral as you progress through the motion.
- Your knees to align over your ankles.
- Your body to remain close to the chair.

AVOID
- Allowing your shoulders to lift up toward your ears.

3 Tuck your tailbone toward the front of the chair, and bend your knees toward your chest. Bend your elbows simultaneously. At the bottom of the movement, extend your elbows and press through your shoulders.

4 Keeping your head in neutral position, press into the chair and lower your legs to return to the starting position. Repeat fifteen times for two sets.

QUICK GUIDE

TARGET
- Shoulder stabilizers
- Triceps

BENEFITS
- Strengthens upper body
- Improves shoulder stability

NOT ADVISABLE IF YOU HAVE
- Shoulder pain
- Neck pain

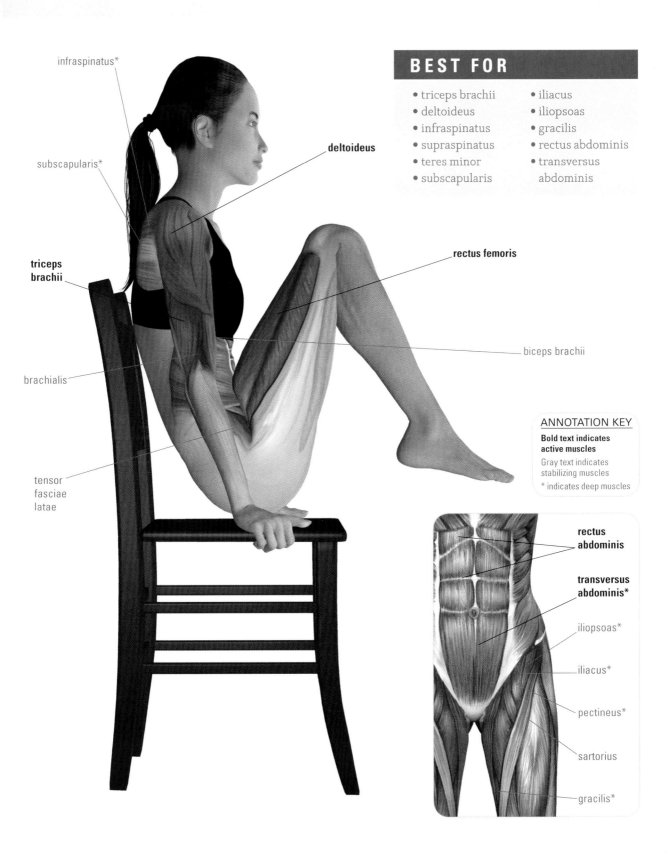

infraspinatus*

subscapularis*

deltoideus

triceps
brachii

rectus femoris

brachialis

biceps brachii

tensor
fasciae
latae

BEST FOR

- triceps brachii
- deltoideus
- infraspinatus
- supraspinatus
- teres minor
- subscapularis
- iliacus
- iliopsoas
- gracilis
- rectus abdominis
- transversus
  abdominis

ANNOTATION KEY

**Bold text indicates
active muscles**

Gray text indicates
stabilizing muscles

* indicates deep muscles

**rectus
abdominis**

**transversus
abdominis***

iliopsoas*

iliacus*

pectineus*

sartorius

gracilis*

PUSH-UP HAND WALK-OVER

CORE STRENGTH

① Start in a plank position with your left hand on the floor and your right on an elevated box or step between four and six inches high.

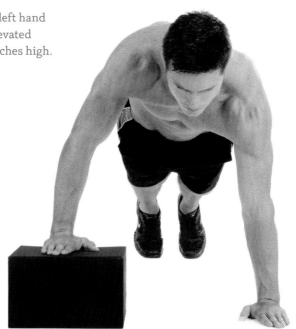

QUICK GUIDE

TARGET
• Total-body strengthening and stabilization

BENEFITS
• Strengthens the pelvic, trunk, and shoulder stabilizers

NOT ADVISABLE IF YOU HAVE
• Shoulder pain
• Back pain
• Neck pain

② Keeping your torso rigid and your legs straight, bend your elbows into a push-up position.

③ Push back up, straightening your elbows to return to the starting position.

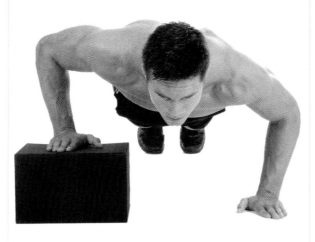

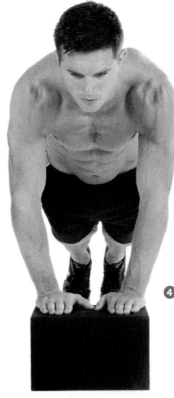

④ Lift your left hand off the floor, and place it beside your right on the top of the box.

BEST FOR

- vastus medialis
- vastus lateralis
- vastus intermedius
- rectus femoris
- gluteus maximus
- pectoralis major
- pectoralis minor
- deltoideus
- triceps brachii
- rectus abdominis
- erector spinae
- trapezius
- latissimus dorsi
- quadratus lumborum

DO IT RIGHT

LOOK FOR
- Your hands to align under your shoulders.

AVOID
- Dipping your shoulders to one side.
- Shifting your hips as your hands "walk."
- Craning your neck.

5 Lift your right hand off the box, placing it on the floor about one shoulder width to the right.

6 Bend your elbows to perform another push-up, this time on the other side of the box.

7 Return to the top of the box and repeat. Perform five push-ups on each side.

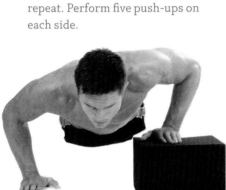

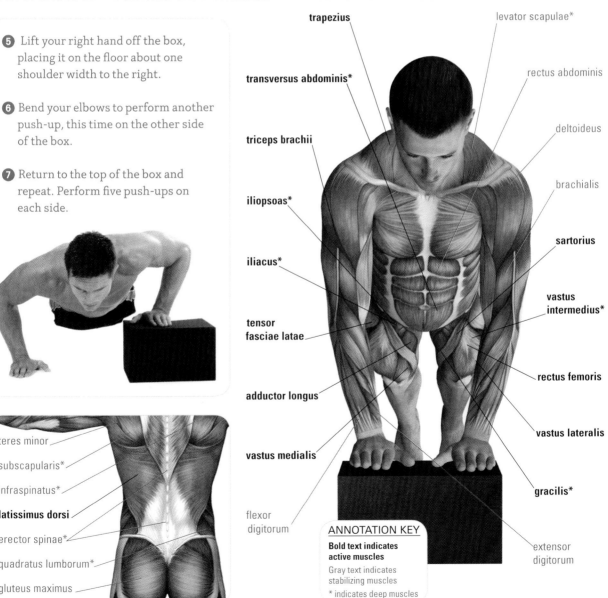

teres minor
subscapularis*
infraspinatus*
latissimus dorsi
erector spinae*
quadratus lumborum*
gluteus maximus

trapezius
transversus abdominis*
triceps brachii
iliopsoas*
iliacus*
tensor fasciae latae
adductor longus
vastus medialis
flexor digitorum

levator scapulae*
rectus abdominis
deltoideus
brachialis
sartorius
vastus intermedius*
rectus femoris
vastus lateralis
gracilis*
extensor digitorum

ANNOTATION KEY
Bold text indicates active muscles
Gray text indicates stabilizing muscles
* indicates deep muscles

OBLIQUE ROLL-DOWN

CORE STRENGTH

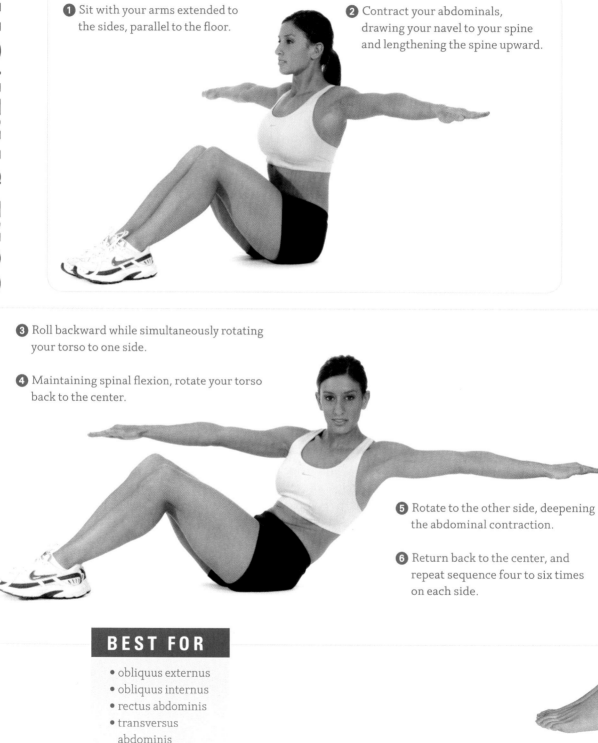

1 Sit with your arms extended to the sides, parallel to the floor.

2 Contract your abdominals, drawing your navel to your spine and lengthening the spine upward.

3 Roll backward while simultaneously rotating your torso to one side.

4 Maintaining spinal flexion, rotate your torso back to the center.

5 Rotate to the other side, deepening the abdominal contraction.

6 Return back to the center, and repeat sequence four to six times on each side.

BEST FOR

- obliquus externus
- obliquus internus
- rectus abdominis
- transversus abdominis

DO IT RIGHT

LOOK FOR
- Your arms to lengthen as you roll down to create opposition throughout the torso.
- Your neck to be relaxed and lengthened to prevent straining.
- Your spine to be articulated while rolling up and down.

AVOID
- Tensing your neck and shoulder muscles.

QUICK GUIDE

TARGET
- Obliques

BENEFITS
- Targets the obliques and abdominals while challenging the ability to maintain the C curve

NOT ADVISABLE IF YOU HAVE
- A herniated disk

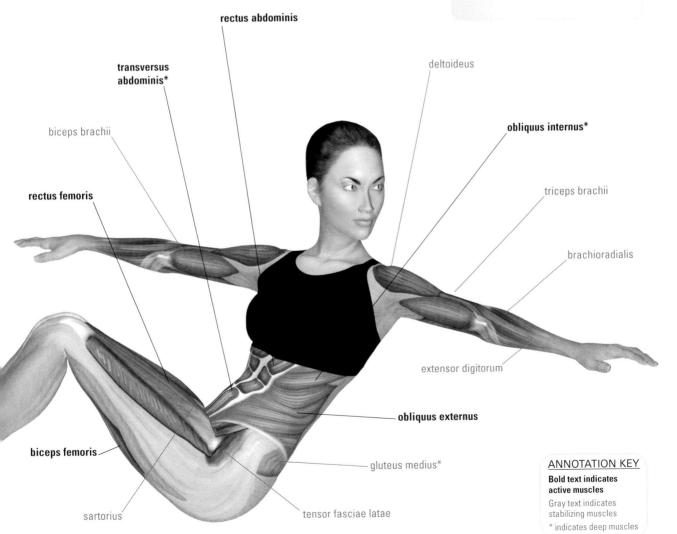

rectus abdominis

transversus abdominis*

deltoideus

biceps brachii

obliquus internus*

rectus femoris

triceps brachii

brachioradialis

extensor digitorum

obliquus externus

biceps femoris

gluteus medius*

sartorius

tensor fasciae latae

ANNOTATION KEY
Bold text indicates active muscles
Gray text indicates stabilizing muscles
* indicates deep muscles

QUADRUPED LATERAL LIFT

CORE STRENGTH

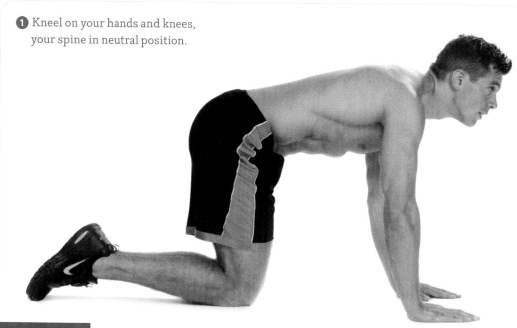

① Kneel on your hands and knees, your spine in neutral position.

BEST FOR

- rectus abdominis
- obliquus internus
- obliquus externus
- transversus abdominis
- gluteus maximus
- gluteus medius
- tensor fasciae latae

② Keep your weight centered and raise your right knee—still bent—out to the side.

③ Raise and lower your leg without moving your hips. Repeat ten times, and then switch legs.

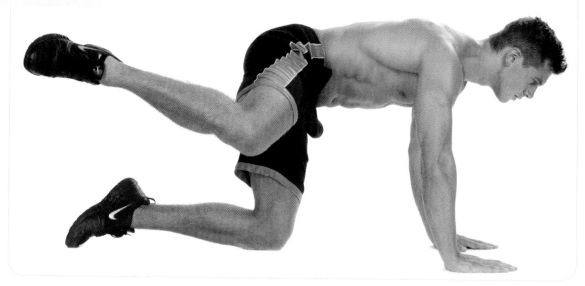

QUICK GUIDE

TARGET
- Core
- Pelvic stabilizers
- Abductor leg muscles

BENEFITS
- Improves pelvic stability
- Strengthens hips and legs

NOT ADVISABLE IF YOU HAVE
- Sharp back pain
- Wrist pain

ANNOTATION KEY
**Bold text indicates
active muscles**
Gray text indicates
stabilizing muscles
* indicates deep muscles

DO IT RIGHT

LOOK FOR
- Your spine to remain neutral, so as to prevent the lower back from sagging.
- Your chin to remain tucked and your head in neutral.
- Your hands to press into the floor and out of the shoulders to keep the shoulders from sinking near the ears.

AVOID
- Lifting the hip as you lift your leg.

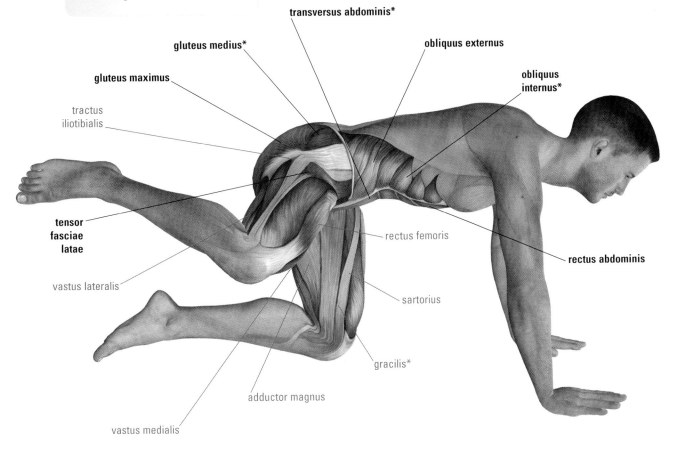

transversus abdominis*

gluteus medius*

obliquus externus

gluteus maximus

obliquus
internus*

tractus
iliotibialis

tensor
fasciae
latae

rectus femoris

rectus abdominis

vastus lateralis

sartorius

gracilis*

adductor magnus

vastus medialis

STANDING KNEE CRUNCH

CORE STRENGTH

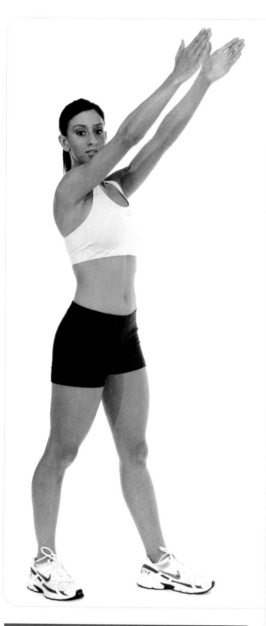

1 Standing tall with your left leg in front of the right, extend your hands up toward the ceiling, your arms straight.

2 Shift your weight onto your left foot, and raise your right knee to the height of your hips. Simultaneously go up on the toes of your left leg, while pulling your elbows down by your sides, your hands making fists. This creates the crunch.

3 Pause at the top of the movement, and then return to the starting position. Repeat the sequence with your right leg as the standing leg. Repeat ten times on each leg.

BEST FOR

- rectus abdominis
- obliquus internus
- obliquus externus
- transversus abdominis
- gluteus maximus
- gluteus medius
- tensor fasciae latae
- piriformis
- iliacus
- iliopsoas
- gastrocnemius
- soleus

QUICK GUIDE

TARGET
• Pelvic and core stabilizers
• Abdominals
• Gluteal muscles

BENEFITS
• Strengthens core
• Strengthens calves and gluteal muscles
• Improves balance

NOT ADVISABLE IF YOU HAVE
• Knee pain

transversus abdominis*
iliacus*
iliopsoas*

triceps brachii
obliquus externus
rectus abdominis
obliquus internus*
vastus intermedius*
rectus femoris
vastus lateralis
sartorius

gluteus medius*
tensor fasciae latae
piriformis
gluteus maximus
vastus medialis
gastrocnemius
soleus

DO IT RIGHT

LOOK FOR
• Your standing leg to be straight as you raise up on your toes.
• Your shoulders to be relaxed as you pull your arms down for the crunch.
• The toes of your raised leg to flex.

AVOID
• Tilting forward as you switch legs.

ANNOTATION KEY
Bold text indicates active muscles
Gray text indicates stabilizing muscles
* indicates deep muscles

FOAM ROLLER CHALLENGE

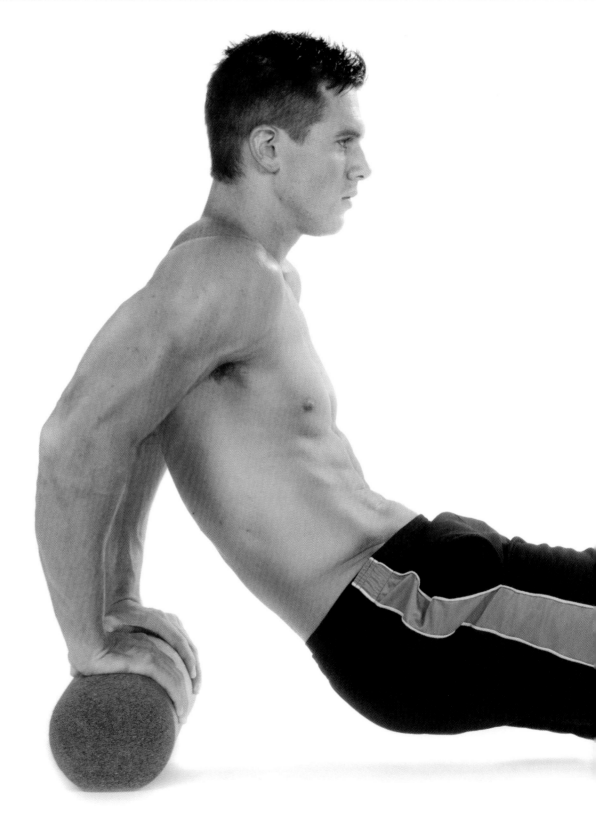

A foam roller is one of the most versatile, affordable, and easy-to-use pieces of fitness training equipment. Rollers come in a variety of sizes, materials, and densities, and they can be used for stretching, strengthening, balance training, stability training, and self-massage. This chapter will provide you with several foam roller exercises that incorporate both core stability and core strengthening, which will add another dimension to your workout.

If you do not have access to a foam roller, you can substitute a pool noodle or a homemade towel roller. To make a towel roller, place two bath towels together, firmly roll them lengthwise, and then wrap the ends with tape. Although a towel roller works well, the dense foam of the roller will provide you with the best results.

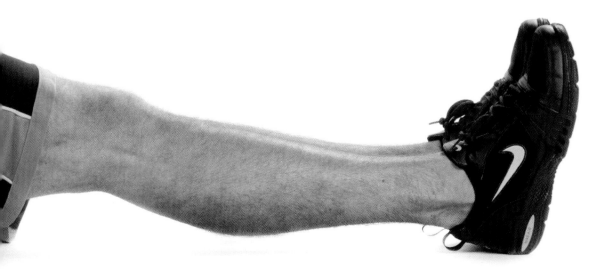

QUADRUPED KNEE PULL-IN

FOAM ROLLER

❶ Place the foam roller on the floor. Kneel on the roller with your hands placed on the floor in front of you. Your hands should be slightly in front of your torso, and your hips should be lifted off your heels.

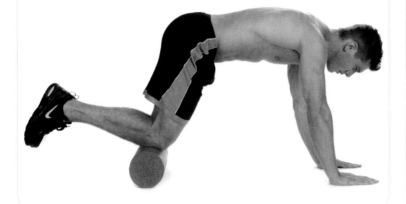

QUICK GUIDE

TARGET
- Triceps
- Abdominals
- Thigh muscles

BENEFITS
- Improves core, pelvic, and shoulder stability

NOT ADVISABLE IF YOU HAVE
- Wrist pain
- Shoulder pain
- Difficulty fully bending your knees

❷ Round out your torso as you pull your knees toward your hands, allowing the roller to move toward your feet. Repeat fifteen times for two sets.

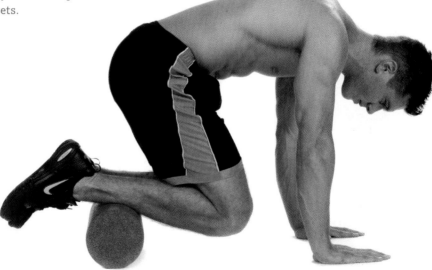

DO IT RIGHT

LOOK FOR
- Your back to round as you draw your knees inward.
- Your head to be relaxed.
- Smooth transitions.

AVOID
- Allowing your shoulders to lift toward your ears.
- Moving your head forward.

MODIFICATION

More difficult: Follow previous instructions, and then bend your elbows into a push-up, straighten, and then roll slowly to the starting position.

ANNOTATION KEY

Bold text indicates active muscles
Gray text indicates stabilizing muscles
* indicates deep muscles

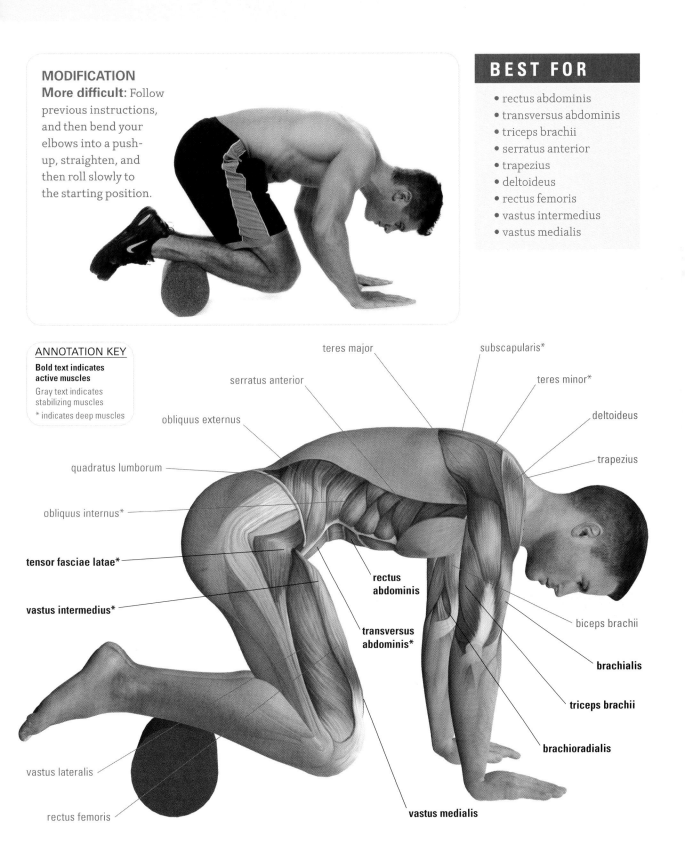

teres major

subscapularis*

serratus anterior

teres minor*

deltoideus

obliquus externus

trapezius

quadratus lumborum

obliquus internus*

tensor fasciae latae*

rectus abdominis

vastus intermedius*

biceps brachii

transversus abdominis*

brachialis

triceps brachii

brachioradialis

vastus lateralis

rectus femoris

vastus medialis

THREAD THE NEEDLE

FOAM ROLLER

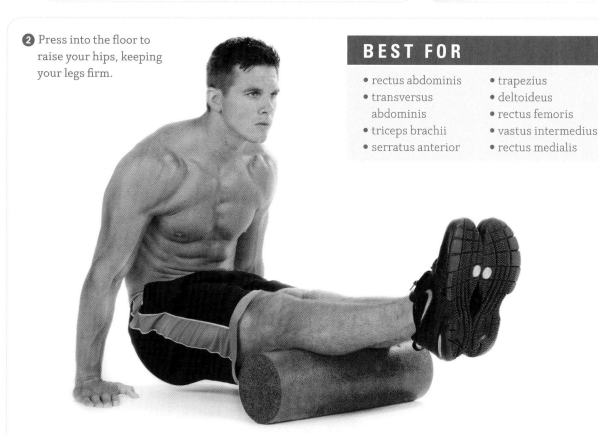

1 Sit on the floor with your legs outstretched in front of you, with the foam roller placed under your knees. Place your hands on the floor to support your torso, your fingers pointing toward your buttocks.

QUICK GUIDE

TARGET
- Abdominals
- Triceps
- Shoulder stabilizers

BENEFITS
- Improves core, pelvic, and shoulder stability

NOT ADVISABLE IF YOU HAVE
- Wrist pain
- Shoulder pain

2 Press into the floor to raise your hips, keeping your legs firm.

BEST FOR

- rectus abdominis
- transversus abdominis
- triceps brachii
- serratus anterior
- trapezius
- deltoideus
- rectus femoris
- vastus intermedius
- rectus medialis

DO IT RIGHT

LOOK FOR
- All movement to happen at the same time.
- Your neck and shoulders to remain relaxed throughout the exercise.

AVOID
- Allowing your shoulders to lift toward your ears.
- Bending your knees as you pull back.

3 Draw your hips backward through your arms, rolling your legs over the roller. Drop your head so that your gaze is directed at your thighs.

4 Roll on the roller back to the starting position, keeping your hips lifted off the floor. Repeat fifteen times.

trapezius
pectoralis minor
pectoralis major
deltoideus
serratus anterior
rectus abdominis
transversus abdominis*
triceps brachii
vastus intermedius*
obliquus internus*
obliquus externus
tensor fasciae latae*
vastus medialis
vastus lateralis
rectus femoris

SINGLE-LEG CALF PRESS

FOAM ROLLER

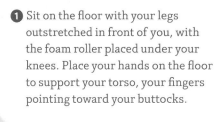

1 Sit on the floor with your legs outstretched in front of you, with the foam roller placed under your knees. Place your hands on the floor to support your torso, your fingers pointing toward your buttocks.

QUICK GUIDE

TARGET
- Triceps
- Shoulder stabilizers
- Abdominals
- Hamstrings

BENEFITS
- Improves core, pelvic, and shoulder stability

NOT ADVISABLE IF YOU HAVE
- Wrist pain
- Shoulder pain
- Discomfort in the back of the knee or knee swelling

2 Press into the floor to lift your hips, keeping your legs firm.

DO IT RIGHT

LOOK FOR
- Your lifted leg to form a long, straight line.
- Your hips to remain elevated throughout the exercise.

AVOID
- Allowing your shoulders to lift toward your ears.
- Bending your knees.
- Bending your elbows.

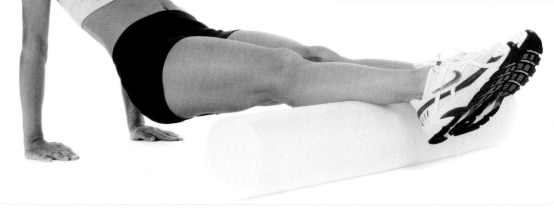

3 Lift one leg off the roller and hold it steady, making sure not to drop your hips.

BEST FOR

- rectus abdominis
- transversus abdominis
- triceps brachii
- serratus anterior
- deltoideus
- biceps femoris
- semitendinosus
- semimembranosus

4 Keep the leg lifted, and press your opposite leg into the roller, drawing your hips back toward your hands.

5 Return to the starting position, rolling your calf muscle along the roller and keeping your lifted leg straight in the air. Repeat fifteen times on each leg.

ANNOTATION KEY
Bold text indicates active muscles
Gray text indicates stabilizing muscles
* indicates deep muscles

adductor magnus

sartorius

vastus medialis

semitendinosus

deltoideus

pectoralis minor*

latissimus dorsi

obliquus internus*

obliquus externus

rectus abdominis

transversus abdominis*

gastrocnemius

plantaris

semimembranosus

biceps femoris

rectus femoris

vastus intermedius*

biceps brachii

brachialis

triceps brachii

brachioradialis

extensor digitorum

gluteus medius*

palmaris longus

gluteus maximus

tibialis posterior*

vastus lateralis

iliopsoas*

iliacus*

tensor fasciae latae*

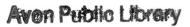
Avon Public Library

ROLLER TRICEPS DIP

FOAM ROLLER

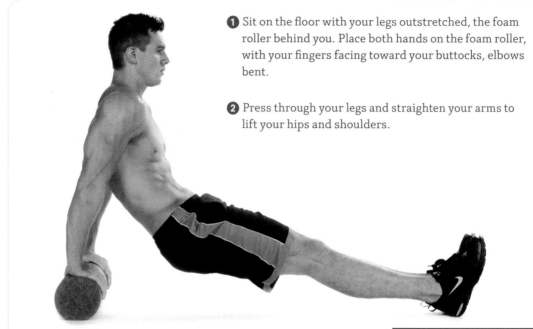

1 Sit on the floor with your legs outstretched, the foam roller behind you. Place both hands on the foam roller, with your fingers facing toward your buttocks, elbows bent.

2 Press through your legs and straighten your arms to lift your hips and shoulders.

3 Keeping your shoulders pressed down away from your ears, bend your elbows and dip your trunk up and down. The foam roller should not move. Repeat fifteen times for two sets.

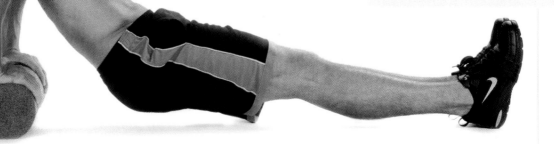

DO IT RIGHT

LOOK FOR
- Your legs to remain firm with your knees straight.
- Your neck and shoulders to remain relaxed throughout the exercise.
- The roller to remain firmly pressed to the floor.

AVOID
- Allowing your shoulders to lift toward your ears.
- Shifting the roller as you move up and down.

BEST FOR

- triceps brachii
- trapezius
- rhomboideus
- deltoideus
- rectus abdominis
- transversus abdominis
- serratus anterior
- biceps femoris
- semitendinosus
- semimembranosus

QUICK GUIDE

TARGET

- Triceps
- Shoulder stabilizers
- Abdominals
- Hamstrings

BENEFITS

- Improves core, pelvic, and shoulder stability

NOT ADVISABLE IF YOU HAVE

- Wrist pain
- Shoulder pain
- Discomfort in the back of the knee or knee swelling

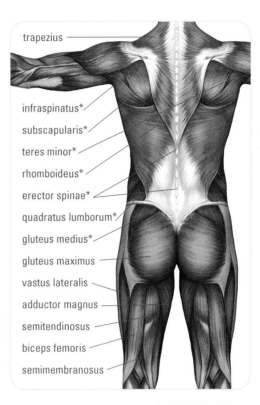

trapezius

infraspinatus*
subscapularis*
teres minor*
rhomboideus*
erector spinae*
quadratus lumborum*
gluteus medius*
gluteus maximus
vastus lateralis
adductor magnus
semitendinosus
biceps femoris
semimembranosus

ANNOTATION KEY

Bold text indicates active muscles

Gray text indicates stabilizing muscles

* indicates deep muscles

deltoideus

triceps brachii

serratus anterior

rectus abdominis

obliquus internus*

transversus abdominis*

obliquus externus

DIAGONAL CRUNCH

FOAM ROLLER

1 Lie lengthwise on the foam roller so that it follows the line of your spine. Your buttocks and shoulders should both be in contact with the roller.

2 With your legs straight and your feet pressed firmly into the floor, extend your arms over your head.

BEST FOR

- rectus abdominis
- transversus abdominis
- triceps brachii
- trapezius
- pectoralis major
- deltoideus
- serratus anterior
- rectus femoris
- vastus intermedius
- biceps femoris
- semitendinosus
- semimembranosus

3 Raise your head, neck, and shoulders as if to do a crunch. Leave your right leg and left arm down on the ground, using your hand for support. Raise your left leg and right arm, and reach for your ankle.

4 Slowly roll down the roller, dropping your raised arm and leg. Repeat on the opposite leg and arm. Repeat fifteen times on each side.

DO IT RIGHT

LOOK FOR
- Your legs to remain firm throughout exercise.
- Your buttocks and shoulders to remain in contact with the roller throughout exercise.

AVOID
- Allowing your shoulders to lift toward your ears.
- Bending the knees.

QUICK GUIDE

TARGET
- Triceps
- Shoulder stabilizers
- Abdominals
- Hamstrings

BENEFITS
- Improves core, pelvic, and shoulder stability

NOT ADVISABLE IF YOU HAVE
- Back pain
- Neck pain

MODIFICATION
More difficult: Keep one leg on the floor for support, and reach both arms toward the raised leg as you crunch up.

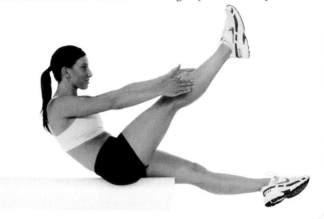

ANNOTATION KEY
Bold text indicates active muscles
Gray text indicates stabilizing muscles
* indicates deep muscles

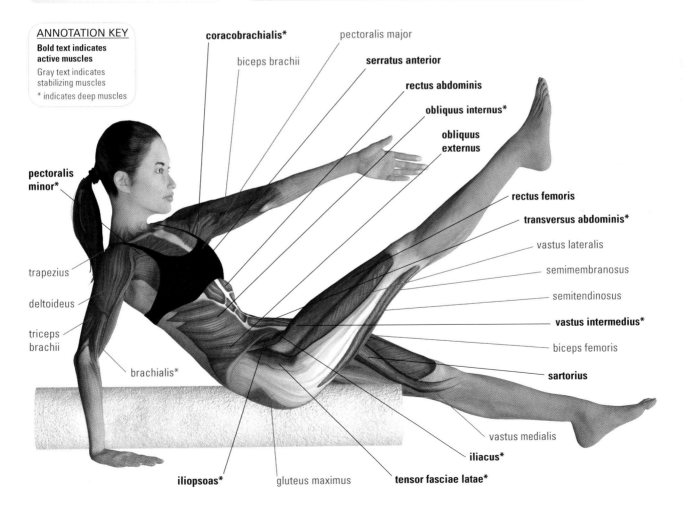

coracobrachialis*

pectoralis major

biceps brachii

serratus anterior

rectus abdominis

obliquus internus*

obliquus externus

pectoralis minor*

rectus femoris

transversus abdominis*

vastus lateralis

semimembranosus

trapezius

semitendinosus

deltoideus

vastus intermedius*

triceps brachii

biceps femoris

sartorius

brachialis*

vastus medialis

iliacus*

iliopsoas*

gluteus maximus

tensor fasciae latae*

ROLLER PUSH-UP

FOAM ROLLER

1 Kneel on the floor with the roller placed crosswise in front of you. Place your hands on the roller with your fingers pointed away from you.

BEST FOR

- rectus abdominis
- transversus abdominis
- triceps brachii
- deltoideus
- pectoralis major
- pectoralis minor
- gluteus maximus
- gluteus medius
- rectus femoris
- biceps femoris

QUICK GUIDE

TARGET
- Triceps
- Shoulder stabilizers
- Abdominals

BENEFITS
- Improves core, pelvic, and shoulder stability

NOT ADVISABLE IF YOU HAVE
- Wrist pain
- Shoulder pain
- Lower-back pain

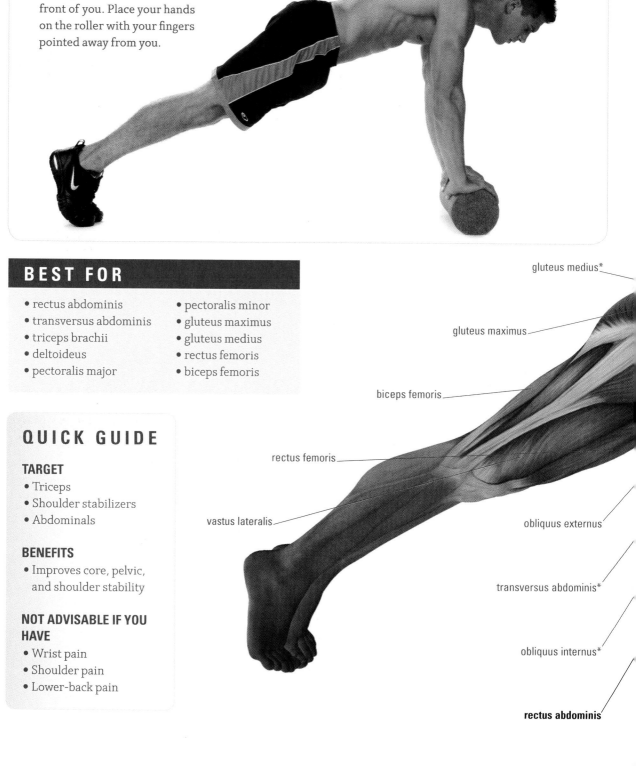

gluteus medius*

gluteus maximus

biceps femoris

rectus femoris

vastus lateralis

obliquus externus

transversus abdominis*

obliquus internus*

rectus abdominis

2 Press into a plank position, lifting your knees and straightening your legs. Keep your hips level with your shoulders, and without allowing your shoulders to sink, bend your elbows and lower your chest to the roller. Avoid any roller movement throughout the motion.

3 Return to the starting position by pressing upward, straightening your elbows, and maintaining a straight spine. Repeat fifteen times for two sets.

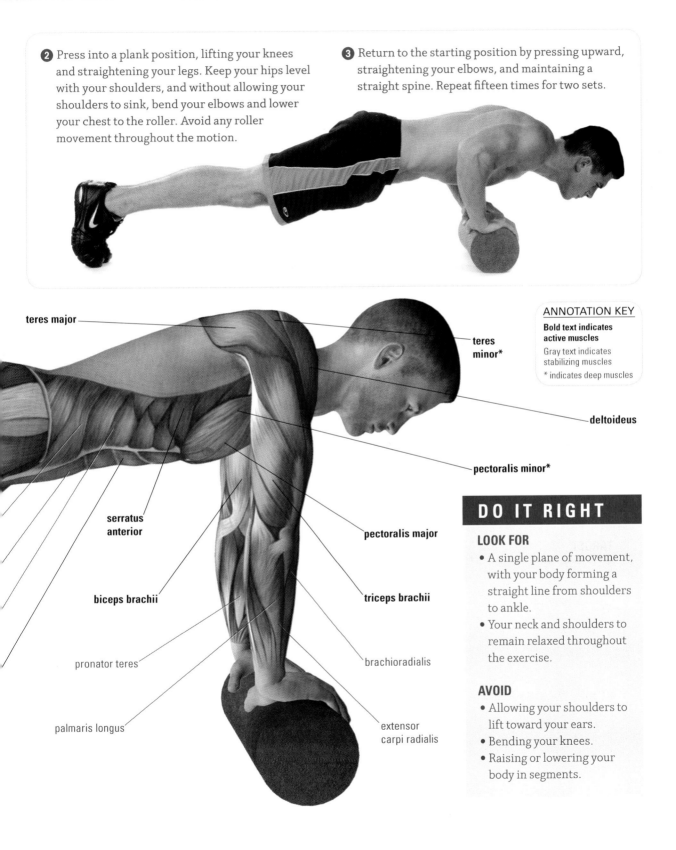

teres major

teres minor*

deltoideus

pectoralis minor*

serratus anterior

pectoralis major

biceps brachii

triceps brachii

pronator teres

brachioradialis

palmaris longus

extensor carpi radialis

ANNOTATION KEY

Bold text indicates active muscles

Gray text indicates stabilizing muscles

* indicates deep muscles

DO IT RIGHT

LOOK FOR

- A single plane of movement, with your body forming a straight line from shoulders to ankle.
- Your neck and shoulders to remain relaxed throughout the exercise.

AVOID

- Allowing your shoulders to lift toward your ears.
- Bending your knees.
- Raising or lowering your body in segments.

SUPINE MARCHES

1 Lie lengthwise on the foam roller so that it follows the line of your spine. Place your arms on the floor by your sides, bending your knees so that your feet rest flat on the floor.

QUICK GUIDE

TARGET
- Triceps
- Abdominals
- Hip flexors
- Quadriceps

BENEFITS
- Improves core and pelvic stability

NOT ADVISABLE IF YOU HAVE
- Lower-back pain
- Neck pain
- Shoulder pain

2 Pointing your toes and keeping the hips from lifting or shifting, raise one knee toward your chest.

3 Switch legs, again being careful not to allow your hips to lift.

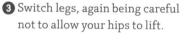

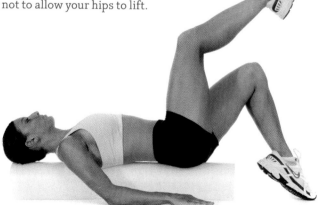

BEST FOR

- rectus abdominis
- transversus abdominis
- obliquus internus
- obliquus externus
- iliacus
- iliopsoas
- sartorius
- biceps femoris
- rectus femoris

4 Repeat fifteen times on each leg as you establish a smooth "marching" rhythm.

DO IT RIGHT

LOOK FOR
- Your legs to remain firm and your toes pointed.
- Your neck and shoulders to remain relaxed throughout the exercise.
- Your hands and forearms to lie flat on the floor.

AVOID
- Allowing your shoulders to lift toward your ears.
- Allowing your hips and lower back to lift off the roller during the movement.

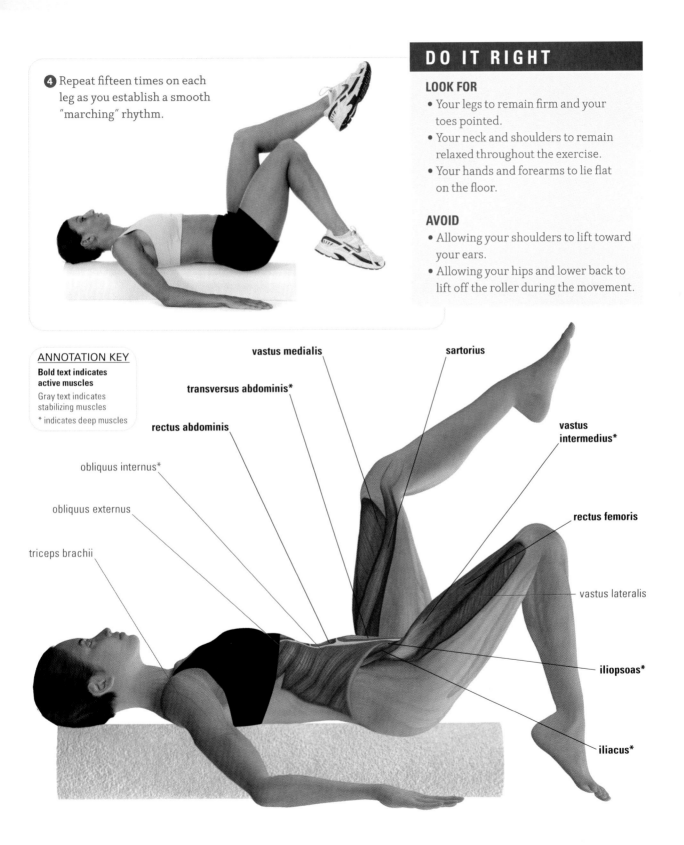

ANNOTATION KEY
Bold text indicates active muscles
Gray text indicates stabilizing muscles
* indicates deep muscles

vastus medialis

sartorius

transversus abdominis*

rectus abdominis

vastus intermedius*

obliquus internus*

rectus femoris

obliquus externus

vastus lateralis

triceps brachii

iliopsoas*

iliacus*

ILIOTIBIAL BAND RELEASE

FOAM ROLLER

❶ Lie on your left side, with the foam roller on the floor and placed under the middle of your thigh. Support your torso with your left forearm on the floor.

❷ Bend your left leg and cross it in front of your right, so that your knee is pointed upward. Place your left foot flat on the floor.

❸ Pulling with your shoulder and pushing with your supporting leg, roll back and forth along the side of your thigh. Adjust the placement of your arm as you make your motion bigger.

❹ Repeat fifteen times on each side.

DO IT RIGHT

LOOK FOR
• Your shoulders to remain relaxed throughout the exercise.
• Your hands and forearms to press firmly into the floor.

AVOID
• Allowing your shoulders to lift toward your ears.

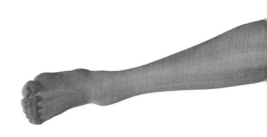

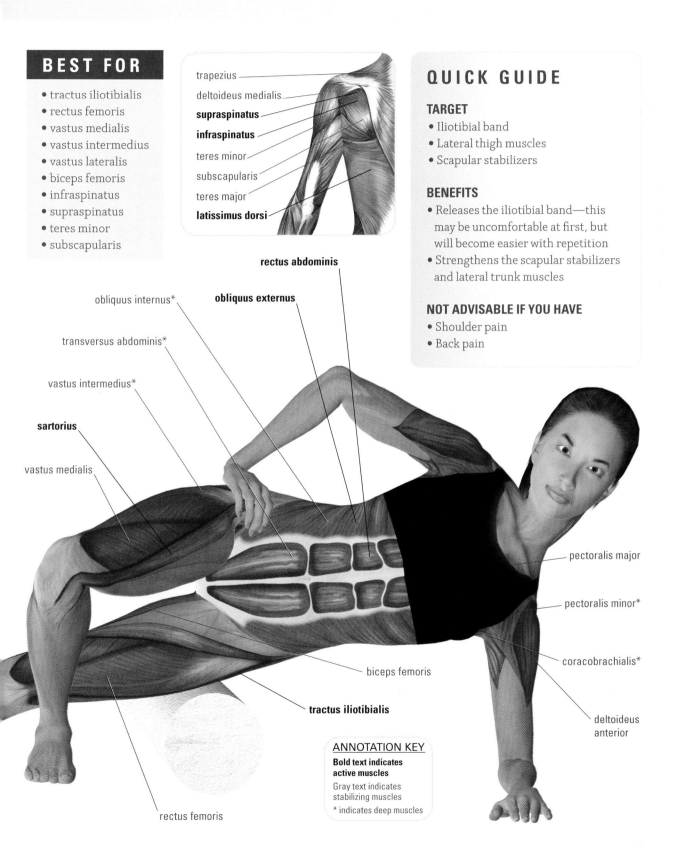

BEST FOR

- tractus iliotibialis
- rectus femoris
- vastus medialis
- vastus intermedius
- vastus lateralis
- biceps femoris
- infraspinatus
- supraspinatus
- teres minor
- subscapularis

trapezius
deltoideus medialis
supraspinatus
infraspinatus
teres minor
subscapularis
teres major
latissimus dorsi

QUICK GUIDE

TARGET
- Iliotibial band
- Lateral thigh muscles
- Scapular stabilizers

BENEFITS
- Releases the iliotibial band—this may be uncomfortable at first, but will become easier with repetition
- Strengthens the scapular stabilizers and lateral trunk muscles

NOT ADVISABLE IF YOU HAVE
- Shoulder pain
- Back pain

rectus abdominis

obliquus internus*

obliquus externus

transversus abdominis*

vastus intermedius*

sartorius

vastus medialis

pectoralis major

pectoralis minor*

coracobrachialis*

biceps femoris

tractus iliotibialis

deltoideus anterior

ANNOTATION KEY
Bold text indicates active muscles
Gray text indicates stabilizing muscles
* indicates deep muscles

rectus femoris

TRICEPS ROLL-OUT

FOAM ROLLER

1 Kneel on the floor, with the foam roller placed crosswise in front of you. Place your wrists on top of the roller, your fingers facing away from you.

DO IT RIGHT

LOOK FOR
- All movement to happen at the same time.
- Your shoulders to remain relaxed throughout the exercise.
- Your feet to press firmly to the floor.

AVOID
- Allowing your shoulders to lift toward your ears.
- Allowing your hips and lower back to drop during the movement.
- Arching your back.

2 Maintaining a neutral spine and making sure not to sink your neck into your shoulders, roll forward on your forearms.

BEST FOR

- rectus abdominis
- transversus abdominis
- triceps brachii
- gluteus maximus
- gluteus medius
- rectus femoris
- biceps femoris
- semitendinosus
- semimembranosus
- erector spinae

3 Continue to roll forward until the roller reaches your elbow. Press into the roller, keeping your hips aligned, and roll back to the starting position. Repeat fifteen times.

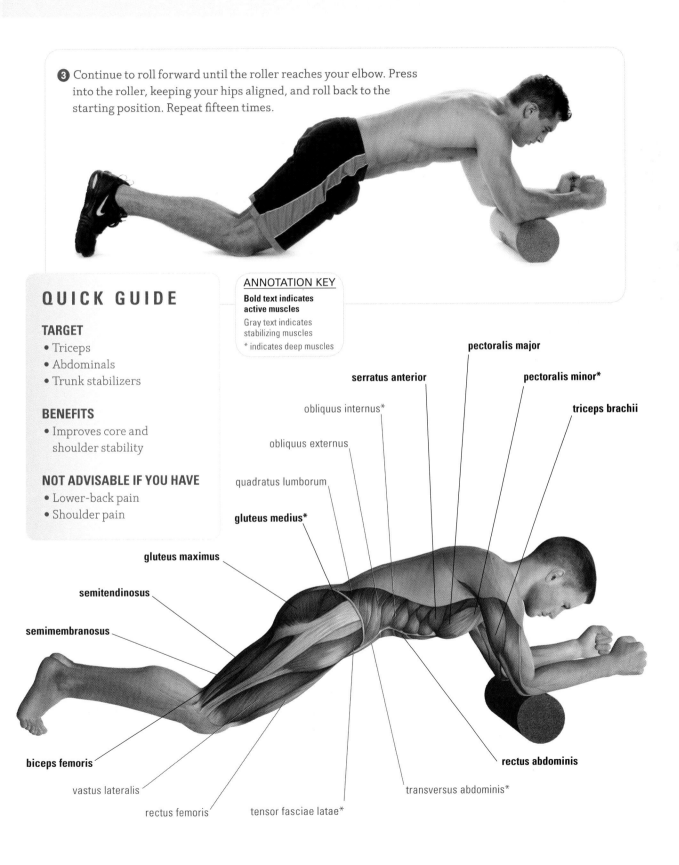

QUICK GUIDE

TARGET
- Triceps
- Abdominals
- Trunk stabilizers

BENEFITS
- Improves core and shoulder stability

NOT ADVISABLE IF YOU HAVE
- Lower-back pain
- Shoulder pain

ANNOTATION KEY
Bold text indicates active muscles
Gray text indicates stabilizing muscles
* indicates deep muscles

pectoralis major

pectoralis minor*

serratus anterior

triceps brachii

obliquus internus*

obliquus externus

quadratus lumborum

gluteus medius*

gluteus maximus

semitendinosus

semimembranosus

biceps femoris

vastus lateralis

rectus femoris

tensor fasciae latae*

transversus abdominis*

rectus abdominis

BRIDGE WITH LEG LIFT I

FOAM ROLLER

1 Lie on your back, with the roller under your shoulders. Your buttocks should be on the floor, with your knees bent, and feet flat on the floor.

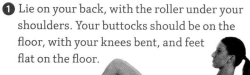

2 Press into the floor with your feet, and bridge up, lifting your hips toward the ceiling until they are parallel to the ground.

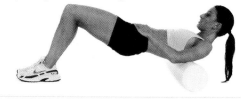

3 Extend your right leg.

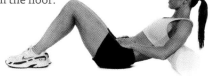

4 Raise your right leg up to the height of your knees. Keeping your leg straight and the roller still, raise and lower your hips.

QUICK GUIDE

TARGET
• Gluteal muscles
• Hamstrings

BENEFITS
• Improves pelvic stabilization
• Strengthens gluteal muscles
• Strengthens hamstrings

NOT ADVISABLE IF YOU HAVE
• Hamstring injury
• Lower-back pain
• Ankle pain

ANNOTATION KEY
Bold text indicates active muscles
Gray text indicates stabilizing muscles
* indicates deep muscles

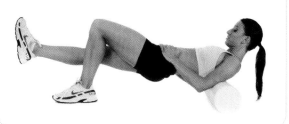

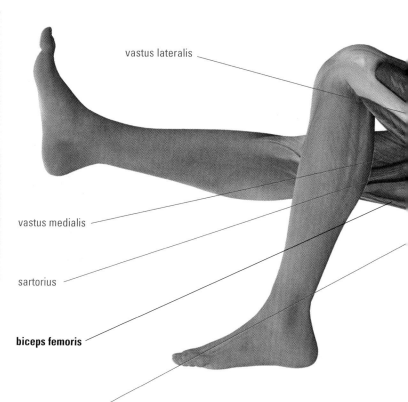

vastus lateralis

vastus medialis

sartorius

biceps femoris

adductor magnus

5 Return to step 2 and repeat step 3 and step 4 with the left leg.

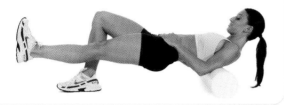

BEST FOR

- rectus abdominis
- transversus abdominis
- obliquus internus
- obliquus externus
- gluteus maximus
- gluteus medius
- vastus intermedius
- rectus femoris
- sartorius
- biceps femoris
- erector spinae

DO IT RIGHT

LOOK FOR
- Your extended leg to remain straight.

AVOID
- Allowing your hips and lower back to drop during the movement.
- Arching your back.

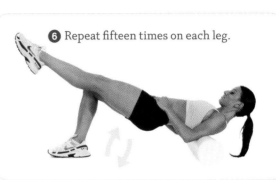

6 Repeat fifteen times on each leg.

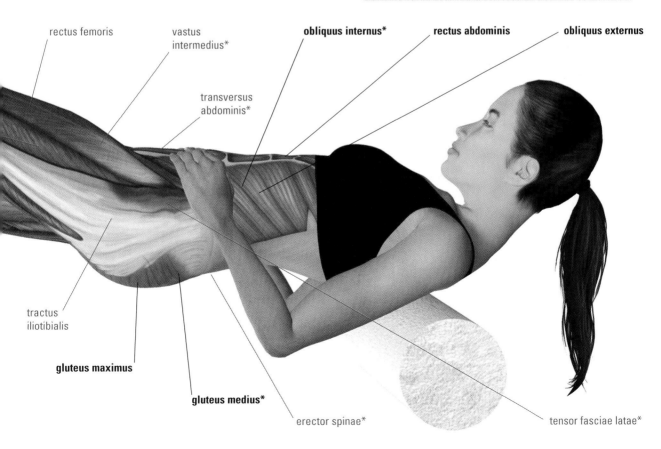

rectus femoris

vastus intermedius*

transversus abdominis*

obliquus internus*

rectus abdominis

obliquus externus

tractus iliotibialis

gluteus maximus

gluteus medius*

erector spinae*

tensor fasciae latae*

BRIDGE WITH LEG LIFT II

FOAM ROLLER

❶ Lie on your back, with the roller under your feet.

❷ Without moving the roller or arching your back, bridge up, and lift your hips into the air.

QUICK GUIDE

TARGET
- Gluteal muscles
- Hamstrings

BENEFITS
- Improves pelvic stabilization
- Strengthens gluteal muscles
- Strengthens hamstrings

NOT ADVISABLE IF YOU HAVE
- Hamstring injury
- Lower-back pain
- Ankle pain

DO IT RIGHT

LOOK FOR
- Your shoulders and neck to remain relaxed throughout the exercise.
- Your extended leg to remain straight.

AVOID
- Allowing your shoulders to lift toward your ears.
- Allowing your hips and lower back to drop during the movement.
- Arching your back.

ANNOTATION KEY
Bold text indicates active muscles

Gray text indicates stabilizing muscles

* indicates deep muscles

vastus lateralis

gluteus maximus

BEST FOR

- rectus abdominis
- transversus abdominis
- obliquus internus
- obliquus externus
- triceps brachii
- gluteus maximus
- gluteus medius
- rectus femoris
- sartorius
- vastus intermedius
- biceps femoris
- semitendinosus
- semimembranosus
- erector spinae

3 Keeping your muscles firm, raise your right leg up to the height of your knees, and straighten your raised leg.

4 Try to keep the roller from moving, and raise and lower your hips while keeping your outstretched leg raised. Repeat fifteen times.

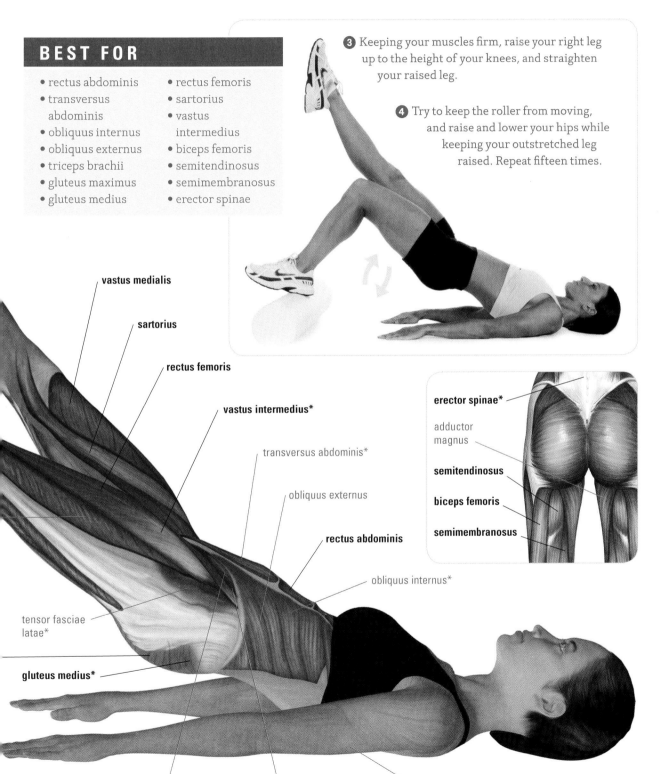

vastus medialis

sartorius

rectus femoris

vastus intermedius*

transversus abdominis*

obliquus externus

rectus abdominis

obliquus internus*

tensor fasciae latae*

gluteus medius*

iliopsoas*

iliacus*

triceps brachii

erector spinae*

adductor magnus

semitendinosus

biceps femoris

semimembranosus

HAMSTRING PULL-IN

FOAM ROLLER

❶ Lie supine on the floor, your knees bent and the roller under your feet.

QUICK GUIDE

TARGET
• Hamstrings
• Gluteal muscles

BENEFITS
• Increases hamstring strength and endurance
• Strengthens gluteal muscles and pelvic stabilizers

NOT ADVISABLE IF YOU HAVE
• Hamstring injury
• Lower-back pain
• Ankle pain

❷ Bridge up, lifting your hips so that they align with the shoulders in a neutral position.

❸ Squeeze your buttocks, and pull your calves in and out as you roll the roller under your feet.

DO IT RIGHT

LOOK FOR
• Your shoulders to remain relaxed throughout the exercise.
• Your body to form a straight line from shoulder to knee.

AVOID
• Allowing your hips and lower back to drop as movement is performed.
• Arching your back.

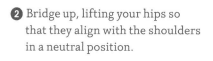
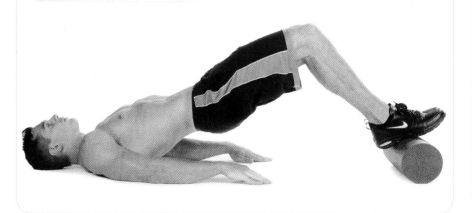

BEST FOR

- rectus abdominis
- transversus abdominis
- gluteus maximus
- gluteus medius
- biceps femoris
- semitendinosus
- semimembranosus
- erector spinae
- quadratus lumborum

4 Repeat fifteen times for two sets.

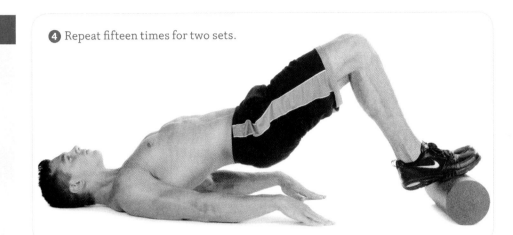

ANNOTATION KEY

Bold text indicates active muscles

Gray text indicates stabilizing muscles

* indicates deep muscles

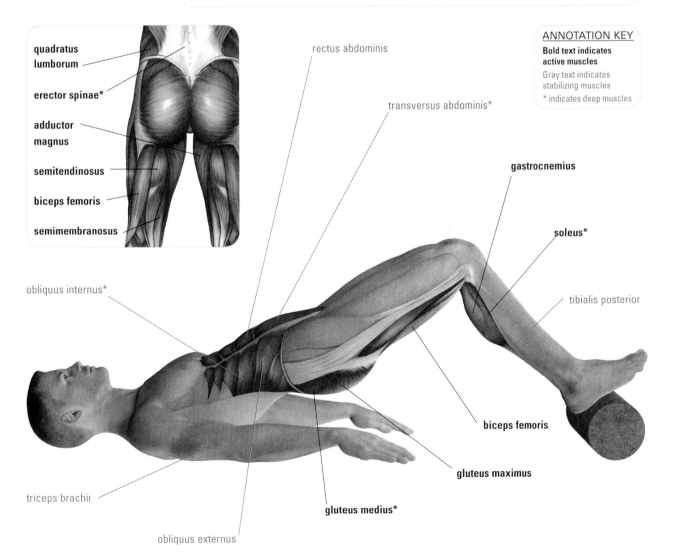

quadratus lumborum

erector spinae*

adductor magnus

semitendinosus

biceps femoris

semimembranosus

rectus abdominis

transversus abdominis*

gastrocnemius

soleus*

tibialis posterior

obliquus internus*

biceps femoris

gluteus maximus

triceps brachii

gluteus medius*

obliquus externus

STRAIGHT-LEG BICYCLE

FOAM ROLLER

1 Lie on your back with the roller placed lengthwise under your spine, your buttocks and shoulders resting on the roller. Place your forearms on the floor on either side of the roller to balance yourself.

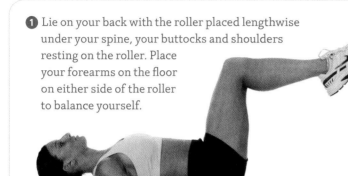

2 Draw your knees up to a tabletop position, forming a 90-degree angle between your hips, thighs, and calves.

QUICK GUIDE

TARGET
- Abdominals
- Thigh muscles

BENEFITS
- Improves pelvic stabilization
- Strengthens abdominals

NOT ADVISABLE IF YOU HAVE
- Lower-back pain
- Neck pain

3 Keeping your back flat, lift your head, neck, and shoulders off the roller. Straighten your right leg and pull your left knee in toward your chest, keeping your head, neck, and shoulders lifted.

BEST FOR

- rectus abdominis
- transversus abdominis
- obliquus internus
- obliquus externus
- triceps brachii
- vastus intermedius
- rectus femoris
- vastus medialis

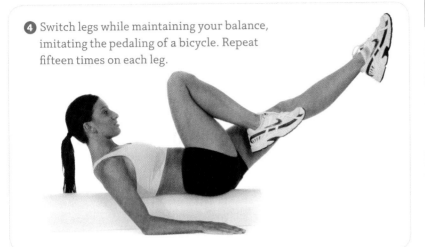

4 Switch legs while maintaining your balance, imitating the pedaling of a bicycle. Repeat fifteen times on each leg.

DO IT RIGHT

LOOK FOR
- Your neck to remain relaxed throughout the exercise.
- Your leg to fully extend during the downward phase of the "pedaling" movement.

AVOID
- Allowing your shoulders to lift toward your ears.
- Lifting your hips and lower back during the movement.

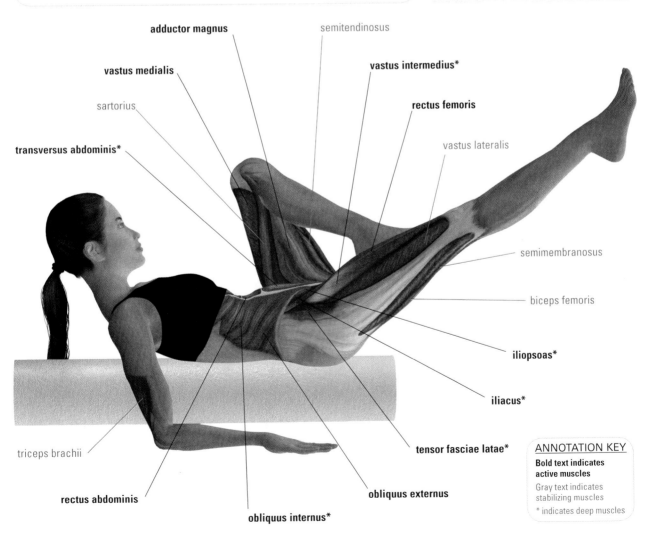

adductor magnus

semitendinosus

vastus medialis

vastus intermedius*

sartorius

rectus femoris

transversus abdominis*

vastus lateralis

semimembranosus

biceps femoris

iliopsoas*

iliacus*

triceps brachii

tensor fasciae latae*

rectus abdominis

obliquus externus

obliquus internus*

ANNOTATION KEY
Bold text indicates active muscles

Gray text indicates stabilizing muscles

* indicates deep muscles

THE DEAD BUG

FOAM ROLLER

① Lie on your back with the roller placed lengthwise under your spine, your buttocks and shoulders resting on the roller. Place your hands and forearms flat on the floor for stabilization. Draw your knees up so that your legs form a tabletop position.

QUICK GUIDE

TARGET
• Abdominals
• Leg muscles

BENEFITS
• Improves pelvic and core stabilization
• Strengthens abdominals

NOT ADVISABLE IF YOU HAVE
• Lower-back pain
• Neck pain

② Lift your head, neck, and shoulders.

③ Press the palms of your hands onto your knees, creating your own resistance as you try to balance. Flex your toes and keep your elbows pulled in to your sides. Hold for ten seconds. Repeat ten times.

DO IT RIGHT

LOOK FOR
• Your hips, thighs, and calves to form a 90-degree angle.
• Your neck to remain relaxed throughout the exercise.
• Your shoulders and buttocks to remain flat on the roller throughout the exercise.

AVOID
• Allowing your shoulders to lift toward your ears.
• Lifting your hips or lower back during the movement.

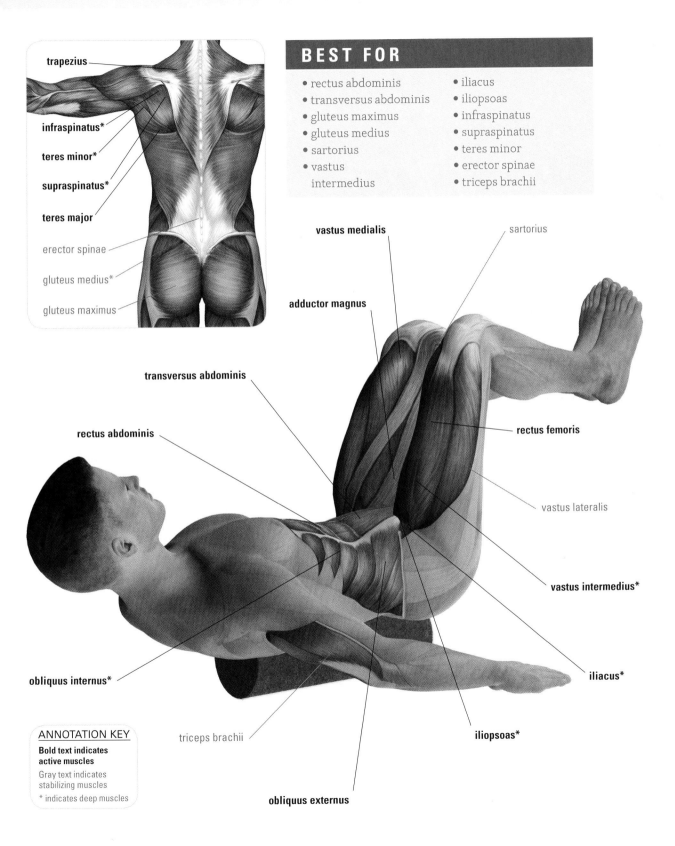

trapezius

infraspinatus*

teres minor*

supraspinatus*

teres major

erector spinae

gluteus medius*

gluteus maximus

BEST FOR

- rectus abdominis
- transversus abdominis
- gluteus maximus
- gluteus medius
- sartorius
- vastus intermedius
- iliacus
- iliopsoas
- infraspinatus
- supraspinatus
- teres minor
- erector spinae
- triceps brachii

vastus medialis

sartorius

adductor magnus

transversus abdominis

rectus abdominis

rectus femoris

vastus lateralis

vastus intermedius*

iliacus*

obliquus internus*

iliopsoas*

triceps brachii

obliquus externus

ANNOTATION KEY
Bold text indicates active muscles
Gray text indicates stabilizing muscles
* indicates deep muscles

SAMPLE WORKOUTS

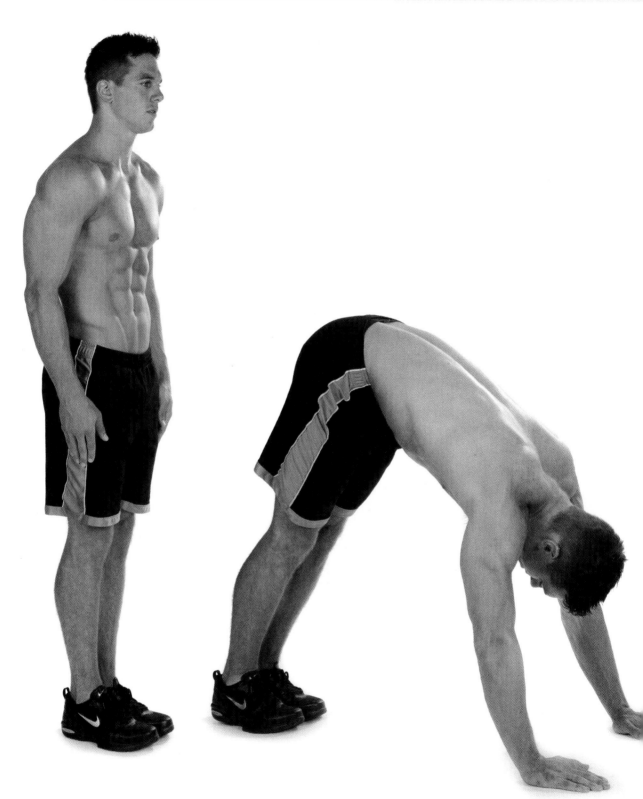

Now that you've familiarized yourself with the core-training exercises, it's time to put them to use. The following three sequences provide you with a comprehensive total-body workout using the exercises that you have learned throughout the book. Each sequence incorporates a few exercises from each section to ensure you a safe and efficient workout. This variety covers and targets the entire body for an overall core activation. These sample workouts will help you get started on a consistent exercise routine, but you can create many additional combinations of the book's exercises. Have fun and mix things up once you feel comfortable with your routine. Each of the sample sequences transitions you to core stability and strengthening. For optimal results, adding a few quick stretches after each exercise sequence will help keep your body lean and supple.

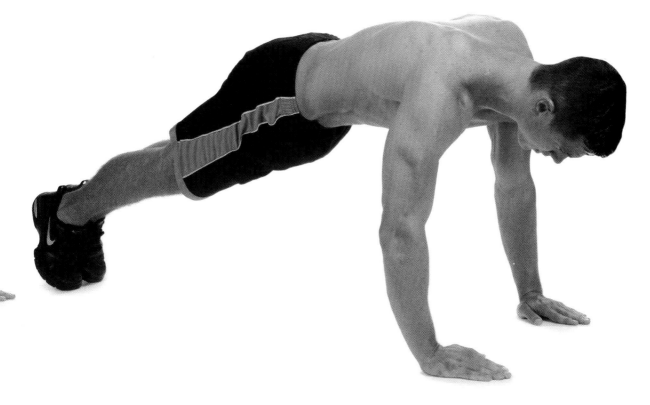

CORE WORKOUT A

SAMPLE WORKOUTS

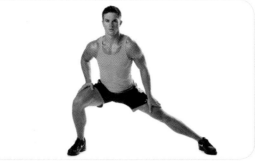

1. Adductor Stretch, page 24

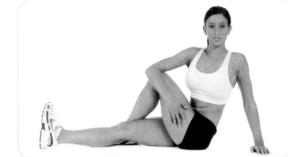

2. Hip Stretch, page 29

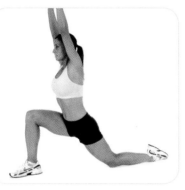

3. Hip Flexor Stretch, page 25

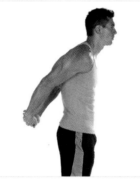

4. Pectoral Stretch, page 21

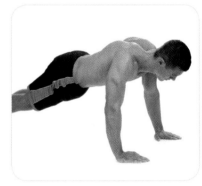

5. Plank Roll-down, page 36

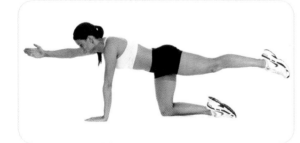

6. Quadruped Leg Lift, page 44

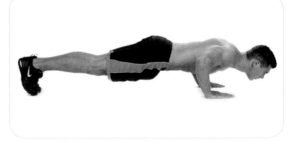

7. Push-up, page 52

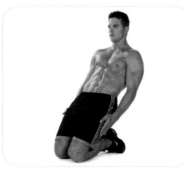

8. Thigh Rock-back, page 42

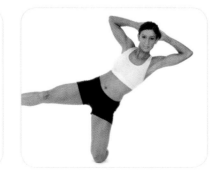

9. Kneeling Side Lift, page 104

10. Oblique Roll-down, page 116

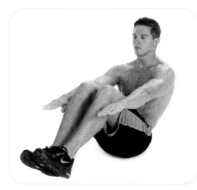

11. Lemon Squeezer, page 90

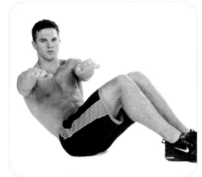

12. Russian Twist, page 94

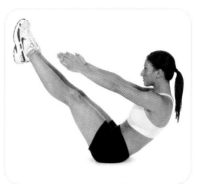

13. V-up, page 92

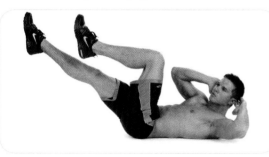

14. Crossover Crunch, page 78

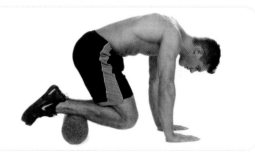

15. Quadruped Knee Pull-in, page 124

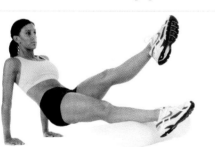

16. Single-Leg Calf Press, page 128

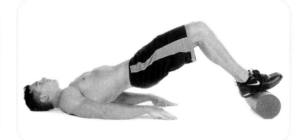

17. Hamstring Pull-in, page 146

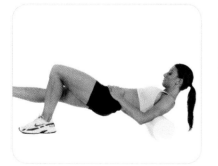

18. Bridge with Leg Lift I,
page 142

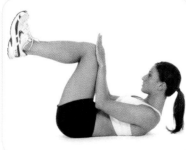

19. Double-Leg Ab Press,
page 68

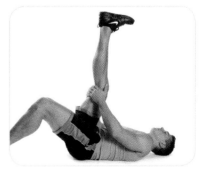

20. Hamstring Stretch,
page 30

CORE WORKOUT B

SAMPLE WORKOUTS

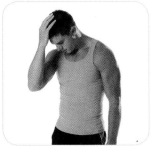

1. Neck Flexion, page 16

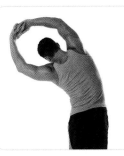

2. Latissimus Dorsi
Stretch, page 19

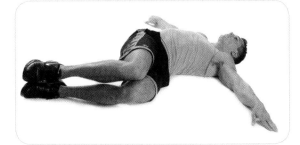

3. Lumbar Stretch, page 27

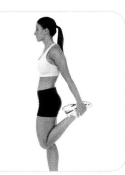

4. Quadriceps Stretch,
page 22

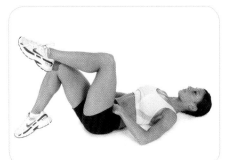

5. Tiny Steps, page 34

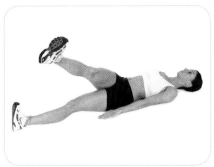

6. Single-Leg Circles, page 40

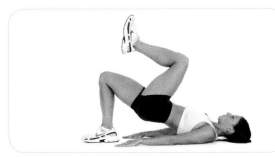

7. Bridge with Leg Lift, page 50

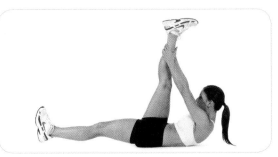

8. Scissors, page 64

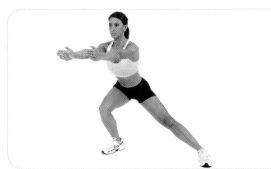

9. Lateral Low Lunge, page 80

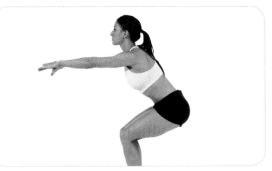

10. Tendon Stretch, page 84

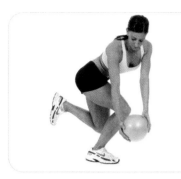

11. Power Squat, page 88

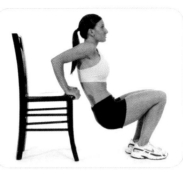

12. Chair Dip, page 54

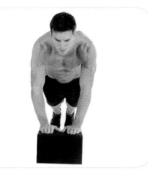

13. Push-up Hand Walk-over,
page 114

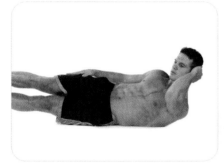

14. Side-Lift Bend, page 98

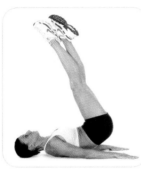

15. Abdominal Hip Lift,
page 108

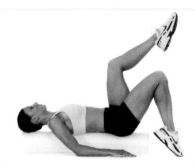

16. Supine Marches, page 136

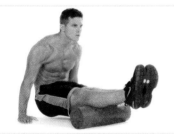

17. Thread the Needle, page 126

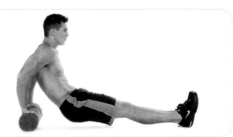

18. Roller Triceps Dip, page 130

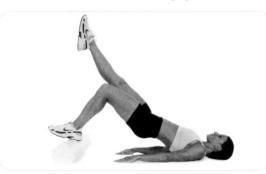

19. Bridge with Leg Lift II, page 144

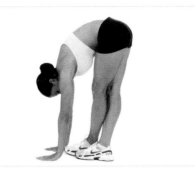

20. Iliotibial Band Stretch, page 23

CORE WORKOUT C

SAMPLE WORKOUTS

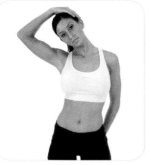
1. Neck Side Bend, page 17

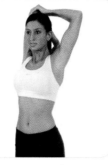
2. Triceps Stretch, page 18

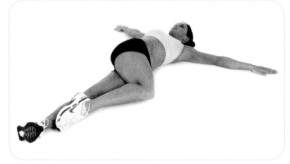
3. Spine Stretch, page 26

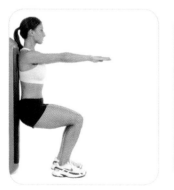
4. Piriformis Stretch, page 28

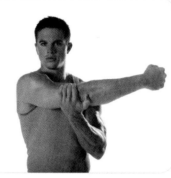
5. Shoulder Stretch, page 20

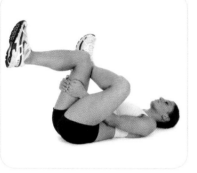
6. Hand-to-Toe Lift, page 58

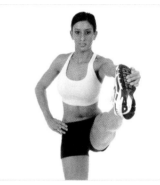
7. Wall Sit, page 60

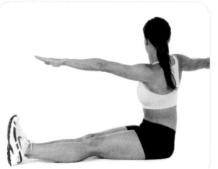
8. Spine Twist, page 38

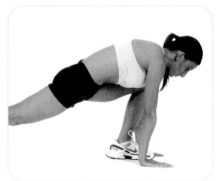
9. High Lunge, page 48

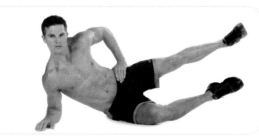
10. Clamshell Series, page 70

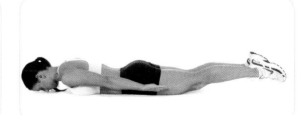
11. Prone Heel Beats, page 72

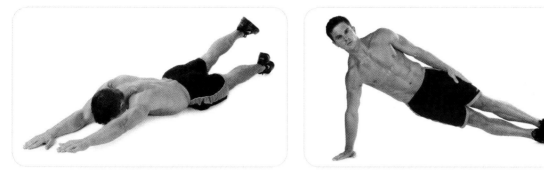

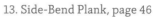

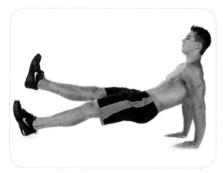

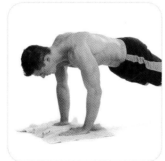

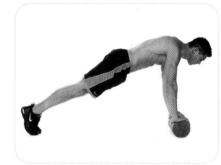

12. Swimming, page 66

13. Side-Bend Plank, page 46

16. Front Plank, page 62

15. Towel Fly, page 56

16. Roller Push-up, page 134

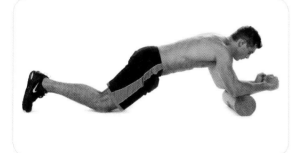

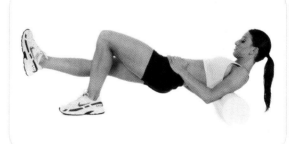

17. Triceps Roll-out, page 140

18. Bridge with Leg Lift I, page 142

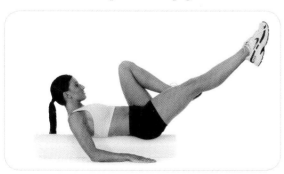

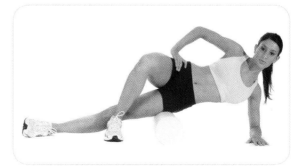

19. Straight Bicycle, page 148

20. Iliotibial Band Release, page 138

CREDITS & ACKNOWLEDGMENTS

All photographs by Jonathan Conklin/Jonathan Conklin Photography, Inc.

Poster illustrations by Linda Bucklin/Shutterstock

Models: Melissa Grant and Michael Radon

All illustrations by Hector Aiza/3D Labz Animation India,
except the insets on pages 12, 13, 16, 19, 21, 24, 25, 26, 27, 28, 29, 31, 35, 37, 43, 47, 49, 53, 55, 57, 61, 63, 69, 71, 72, 83, 91, 103, 107, 111, 113, 115, 121, 139, 145, 151 by Linda Bucklin/Shutterstock

ACKNOWLEDGMENTS

I would like to thank all who helped me prepare this book: To my husband, Tom, for being patient on the weekends, and my clients who diligently proofed the exercises with me. Their hard work and dedication made this book a pleasure to create. I hope you enjoy this book as much as I did putting the material together.

The author and publisher also offer thanks to those closely involved in the creation of this book: Moseley Road president Sean Moore; editor/designer Amy Pierce; art director Brian MacMullen; editorial director/designer Lisa Purcell; and editorial assistant Rebecca Axelrad.